NATURAL
PAINKILLERS

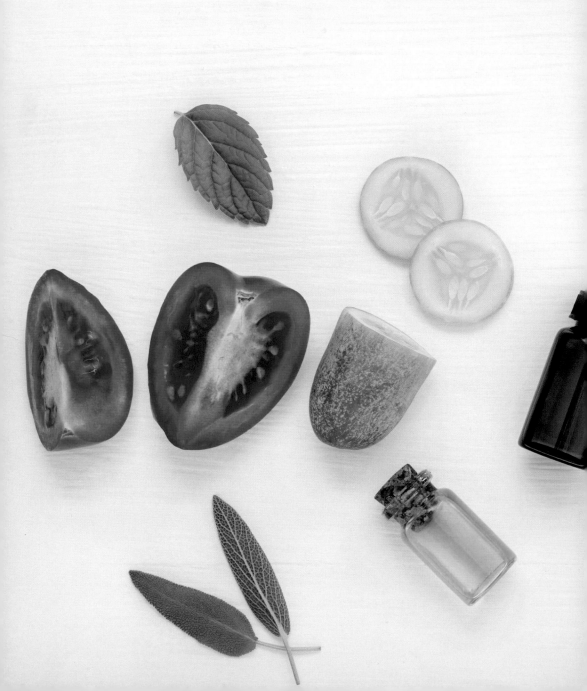

Dr Yann Rougier
& Marie Borrel

NATURAL PAINKILLERS

LEARN HOW TO GET RID OF PAIN THROUGH DIET, EXERCISE, BREATHING TECHNIQUES, MASSAGE, AND MORE!

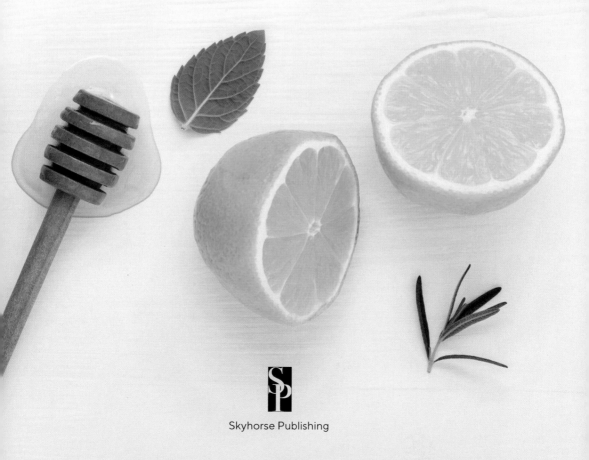

Skyhorse Publishing

PLEASE NOTE
The author and publisher cannot accept any responsibility for misadventure
resulting from the practice of any of the principles and techniques set out in this
book. This book is not intended as guidance for the treatment of serious health
problems; please take note of any cautionary advice given, and refer to a medical
professional if you are in any doubt about any aspect of your condition.

AVAILABILITY OF REMEDIES
If you are unable to obtain any of the recommended remedies in the form
specified, seek advice from a suitably qualified medical professional for
guidance on appropriate substitutes.

CONTENTS

INTRODUCTION

It twinges, it burns, it pounds, it pierces, it stings, it throbs ... in short, it hurts! Nobody is immune. No one goes through life without pain – at best unpleasant, at worst unbearable – intruding at times. Whether it's a migraine, toothache, joint pain, a bad back or stomach ache, pain is part of our lives and, with the best will in the world, we can't eradicate it.

We were all born with a cry that paediatricians agree today reveals the suffering felt by fetuses as they push their way through the birth canal, then, as newborns, swallow their first breath of air as their lungs unfold. Did we come into the world in pain? It's quite likely. We have no memory of this painful feeling, yet it forms the backdrop against which all our future pains resonate, whether slight or intense.

Medical management of pain is fairly recent. Since the mid-twentieth century, new therapeutic approaches have made it possible to suppress suffering in extreme situations, especially for people in the last phases of incurable disease. But what about everyday pain, of the sort that disrupts our wellbeing without endangering our lives? Usually, we 'kill' it with over-the-counter analgesics (aspirin, paracetamol, ibuprofen and so on). However, such drugs are not without risks. They may be suitable for occasional use – a sprained wrist that prevents you writing for a few days or toothache that requires a trip to the dentist – but when the pain intensifies or sets in for a longer period, things are different. The effect of medication decreases when it's taken regularly, and long-term use can produce undesirable side-effects.

So what can be done? Do we make a dive for the first drugs we come across with no regard for the risks, or do we try, stoically, to simply tolerate the pain? The best course of action lies between the two. Pain is, first and foremost, a message that we need to listen to. It's a signal to us that 'something' is wrong with our body, whether it's a simple splinter in the finger, gastric inflammation or a slipped disc. Incidentally, it's worth noting that the intensity of the pain may not correlate with the severity of the problem, although it will certainly determine the urgency with which we deal with it.

It's important, therefore, to hear the message before trying to numb the pain; otherwise the problem may continue to develop silently. In doing so, we also need to be aware of the origin of the pain in order to deal with the cause: extract the splinter, relieve the inflammation or whatever. Take a simple toothache. This is usually a sign that a cavity is forming in the tooth dentine and is getting close to the pulp chamber housing the nerve. Painkillers may get rid of the pain, but they won't prevent decay from continuing on its merry way. So be careful not to put the cart before the horse!

Once the underlying cause has been identified, suffering is no longer necessary. The signal has been heard and we can act. Then comes the second step: finding a painkilling solution suitable for the problem. And the choice is vast! In addition to drugs, which can be reserved for emergencies or for severe pain, traditional medicine offers a wealth of safe and effective painkilling products and methods.

There's herbal medicine, of course, as well as the essential oils extracted from various plants. But they are far from the only recourse. Staples such as clay and bicarbonate of soda (baking soda) can control certain types of pain. Making changes to your diet can be effective for recurrent inflammatory pain. Add breathing exercises, anti-stress techniques, yoga and massage to all this and you have an arsenal of weapons with which to combat all (or almost all) the usual pains of everyday life, without running the slightest risk to your body. Let's face it: why deprive yourself of pain relief!

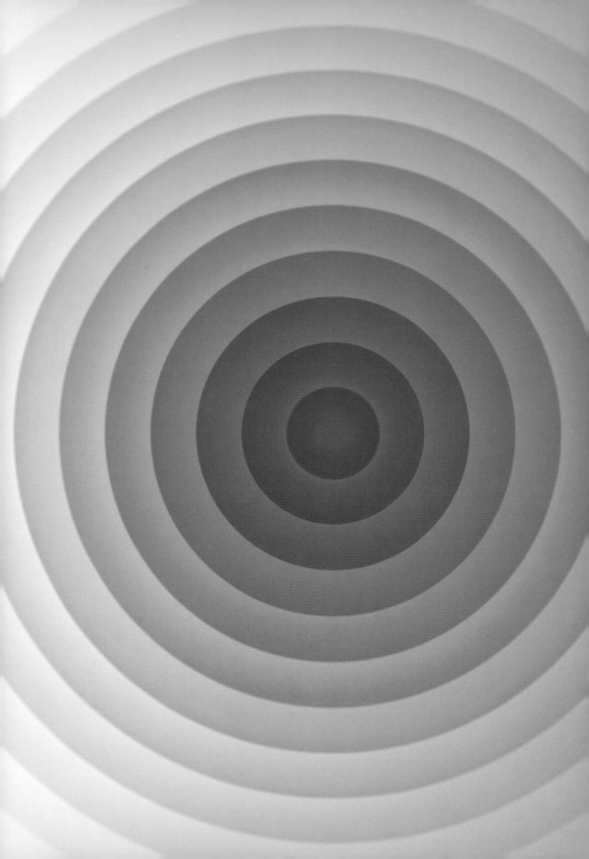

HOW PAIN IS TRANSMITTED

Pain is an 'enemy' that comes in many guises, but we can only fight effectively what we know. It's important, therefore, to gain a better understanding of this multi–faceted phenomenon. There are many types of pain, including external pain due to superficial injury; internal pain resulting from damage to or dysfunction of an internal organ; pain with a strong psychological element; pain devoid of a detectable physiological origin; and phantom pain.

EXTERNAL OR INTERNAL?

Most types of pain can be classified in two broad categories – external and internal. The most common type of pain is due to an activation of sensory receptors in the skin caused by external factors. Our skin is not just 'wrapping paper', a covering that protects us from external aggression; it's also a major interface between our inner world and the one around us.

The skin contains thousands of sensors that enable us to feel hot or cold, dry or wet, rough or smooth, firm or soft. It's also thanks to these receptors that we feel certain types of pain, like the sort that hits when you inadvertently put your hand on a scorching iron. Here, pain serves a very clear purpose: it's the painful sensation that prompts you to remove your hand quickly to escape danger.

This type of pain is mainly related to superficial skin damage (a scratch or cut, for example), but also relates to damage that occurs in the deeper layers of the skin, such as bumps and bruises. Burns cause pain of the same order, regardless of whether – depending on the degree of gravity – they affect only the surface of the skin or are more invasive.

The second category of pain is that which has an internal origin. This kind of pain is indicative of organ damage, deep tissue inflammation or joint problems. Let's get one thing straight: organs are actually pain-free. The pain signal is emitted by the surrounding tissues, which are richly supplied with nerves. In fact, ordinarily, we don't feel our internal organs. Of course, we're conscious of our heart beating or our lungs expanding, but we're unaware of our kidneys, liver, spleen or pancreas – to the extent that most of us have a hard time knowing exactly where in our body those organs are located.

An injury needs be severe for us to perceive pain in an organ – an ulcer perforating the stomach or the wall of the heart beginning to deteriorate due to lack of oxygen, for example. But, even in such cases, it's not always at the level of the organ itself that we feel pain. A heart attack can cause pain in the chest, in the wrist or on the inner side of the left arm. Pain related to gallstones is often felt in the back. Why? Because pain signals relating to external (skin) and internal (organ) causes are transmitted together to the brain, through the same neural pathways. The brain tends to 'confuse' the two and to treat deep pain as though it were superficial.

UNCLASSIFIABLE PAIN
- Some pain doesn't have a tangible cause. This is the pain that's felt in the area of a limb that has been amputated, or by sufferers of diseases such as fibromyalgia. In these cases, there's no internal or external stimulus causing the pain.
- The sensation is the result of a dysfunction of the nervous system, which transmits pain devoid of meaning. The pain exists by and for itself, without carrying any sort of signal that would allow the sufferer to deal with the root of the problem.
- This sort of pain is more difficult to eradicate – but, fortunately, is also much rarer.

ONE STIMULUS, BILLIONS OF NEURONS

In all cases, pain takes the same pathways. These are very complex, but they follow more or less the same pattern. Here's a simplified overview. Once activated, the internal and external receptors send an electrical impulse along the nerves. This information reaches the spinal cord, then travels along a sensory pathway known as the spinothalamic tract to finally reach the thalamus, a large 'marshalling yard' for nerve signals in the brain. Here, the pain is 'coloured' by the tone of previous suffering and the emotions that accompany it. This is where 'the pain' becomes 'your pain'. In the final stage, the signal reaches the cerebral cortex of the brain, where it's decrypted. Ouch! That whole process lasted only a few thousandths of a second.

This schematic journey is regulated by additional systems. First, there's a complex device known as the 'gate control', which is able to modulate the intensity of the signal by letting some bits of information pass and diverting others. It intervenes most notably in the case of chronic pain.

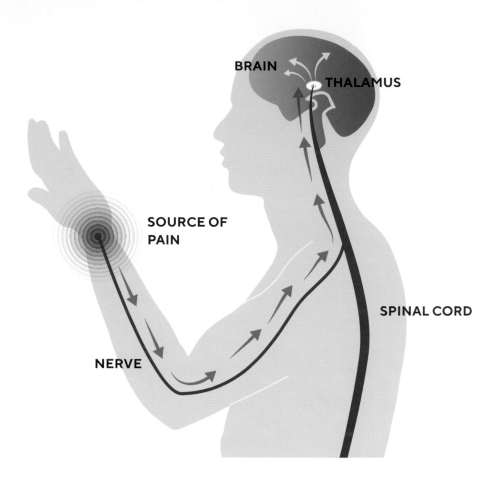

BRAIN

THALAMUS

SOURCE OF
PAIN

SPINAL CORD

NERVE

INVALUABLE NEUROTRANSMITTERS

Electrical impulses travel through the nervous system and the brain with the help of chemicals known as neurotransmitters. These chemicals allow the impulses to pass between nerve cells, or neurons. Neurotransmitters are produced by the body and serve as a 'vehicle' for information circulating in the brain. Each neurotransmitter enables the dissemination of a particular type of information. Some, such as acetylcholine, stimulate the delivery of pain signals, while others, such as endorphins, slow down and dull the signals. Anything that can cause the body to produce more of the latter than the former will help to ease pain. Better management of stress and negative emotions, in particular, will improve the effectiveness of these body-produced painkillers.

MY PAIN, YOUR PAIN, THEIR PAIN

The brain triggers the body's pain-modulation devices under the influence of factors external to the sensation itself, such as stress, anxiety and fear. This explains why each of us experiences pain differently, but it's also the reason that we can combat pain using anti-stress techniques such as relaxation and breathing exercises.

The same pain may be experienced differently by different people. Take the example of a violent migraine. A person whose mother or father suffered a stroke will feel a level of anxiety that will accentuate the painful sensation. Each of us has a particular sensitivity to certain types of pain, which will feel unbearable for us because of our previous experiences.

In any case, everyone will express the pain they feel in words that make sense only to them. It's extremely difficult to describe pain, or even to give a clear indication of its intensity, especially since each of us has our own 'pain threshold' – a level at which pain will be experienced as unbearable. To return to the migraine example: one person may endure it without too much trouble, whereas another may be unable to carry out their daily tasks, their forehead or temples besieged by searing, throbbing pain.

As you can see, pain is a very private experience and difficult to share, which is all the more reason to try to take care of it yourself. But that approach requires the taking of some precautions.

FEELING DIFFERENT

Pain also has a social dimension. In some parts of the world, pain has a ritual or rite-of-passage dimension that allows it to be transcended. In Malaysia, for example, at certain religious festivals, Tamils inflict pain on themselves that to us would seem difficult to bear. In Africa, pain is considered a necessary part of a boy's rite of passage from childhood to adulthood. In the Bible, pain is explained as a consequence of original sin. In any case, giving pain meaning makes it easier to tolerate.

ASKING QUESTIONS OF EACH PAIN SENSATION

Whatever route pain takes, it's important for you to ask certain questions in order to understand how serious the problem is and take urgent action if required, as pain may indicate a potentially serious underlying problem. In the case of a burn or sprain, there's no need to worry: the origin of the pain will be clear and localized. But this isn't true of many types of common everyday pain. A sore throat, for example, may indicate a simple irritation or a serious infection (tonsillitis, for example). That's why, before you begin to treat pain, it's best to ask certain questions:

- Did the pain appear suddenly or gradually?

- Is it recurring?

- Is it associated with a fever?

- Did any other symptoms – nausea, constipation, a stuffy or runny nose, changes in sight or hearing, swelling or rashes – appear at the same time?

If the pain is straightforward, comes on suddenly and isn't accompanied by a fever or any other symptoms, there's no problem; you can treat it on your own. If you suffer from chronic or recurrent pain, such as rheumatism or migraines, the origin of which has been previously confirmed, you can also treat it yourself. But if you have any doubts, don't hesitate to consult your doctor. It's better to be reassured about 'nothing' than to let pain drag on when it may be concealing a more serious problem (see pages 122–3).

Once these factors have been clearly established, you'll be able to choose what suits you from the many natural treatments available, which, at least, will bring you some welcome relief and, at best, will eliminate the pain.

ACUTE AND CHRONIC PAIN

Beside the question of the cause of pain, which should always be determined, there's one particular question you should ask yourself: is the pain transitory ('acute') or long-lasting ('chronic')? The pain-management strategies to be implemented will differ depending on the answer.

Pain caused by a burn or bruise is acute and will vanish on its own as the injured tissue heals. Treatment, which is designed to 'support' and boost this recovery, can therefore also be temporary. The situation is different, though, when pain becomes chronic. When osteoarthritis damages certain joint tissues, the body doesn't know how to repair the damage itself. Pain management therefore needs to be more generalized. In addition to short-term treatments aimed at relieving the affected joint (such as poultices, massages and plant-based remedies), making small changes to your daily lifestyle (such as anti-stress techniques and diet) will enable you to cope with the pain more easily, limit its scope and reduce flare-ups. With chronic pain, you'll need to act on several levels at the same time, even beyond the physical crisis itself, by establishing daily habits designed to help your condition.

*Is your natural arsenal ready?
Then it's time to begin your journey to sure
and lasting pain relief.*

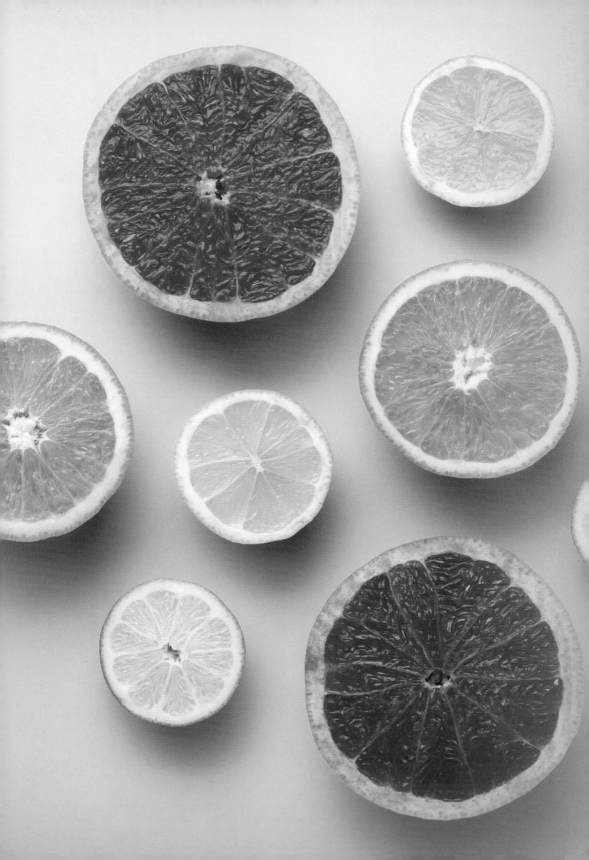

A PAIN-FIGHTING DIET

With pain, whatever its nature and cause, there's often underlying inflammation. Take a simple sprain, for instance. When the ligaments that support the bones are injured as a result of impact or a sudden forceful movement, inflammation occurs so that blood can flow to the damaged tissue, helping to nourish and repair it. This happens in most types of painful injury. Inflammation is involved in toothache, rheumatic pain, migraines and indigestion.

Inflammation isn't your enemy. Indeed, it's often essential to recovery, which then eliminates the pain. It's one of the tools the body uses to repair itself. However, inflammation often lasts longer than it needs to and must be reduced in order to relieve pain. Diet can be one of the best means of doing this, especially in cases of chronic pain, which sufferers have to learn to live with on a daily basis.

TOO MUCH ACIDITY - MORE PAIN

The body is made up of almost 70 per cent water. As well as the liquids that circulate in the body, such as blood and lymph, our cells are immersed in a liquid environment, where all their exchanges occur: they feed on it, draw the oxygen they need from it and eject their waste into it. For cells to function in the right conditions, it's important that this liquid is not too acidic. A balance is permanently established in our body between acidity and alkalinity, and it's essential for all our tissues that this balance remains stable and that the level of acidity doesn't increase.

Acidity is mainly the result of what we eat. When digested and assimilated, some foods – particularly red meat, refined cereals and sugar – cause the production of acidic substances. Conversely, others – notably fresh vegetables and a lot of fruits – contain minerals that resist acids and make them alkaline. This being the case, there are a few simple rules that anyone suffering from chronic or recurrent pain should integrate into their daily life.

Just to be clear – the contents of your plate won't alone be sufficient to suppress intense pain. But all painkilling remedies will be most effective when the level of acidity in the body is balanced. And that's without taking into account the fact that excess acidity in the body encourages the appearance of certain painful disorders, such as headaches, bloating and joint pain. By adapting your daily diet to make it more alkalizing, you can avoid such problems.

IT'S ALL ABOUT pH

The acidity of an environment is calculated using pH (hydrogen potential). The pH of a neutral environment (neither acidic nor alkaline) is around 7, on a scale of 1 to 14. Below a level of 7, an environment becomes acidic; above 7, it's alkaline. Our internal environment should stay within a fairly narrow range (between 7.36 and 7.44), in other words, very slightly alkaline – but only very slightly! Very often, however, it's fairly acidic.

pH SCALE

The pH scale measures how acidic or alkaline a substance is. Pure water, for example, is neutral, with a value of 7, whereas battery acid would be 0 and household bleach around 13.5.

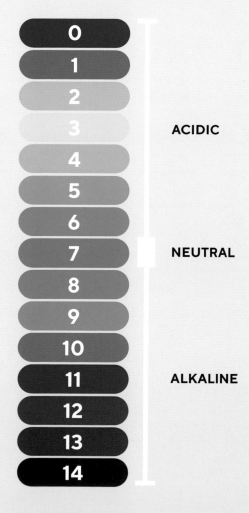

0
1
2
3   ACIDIC
4
5
6
7   NEUTRAL
8
9
10
11   ALKALINE
12
13
14

8 RULES OF A PAIN-FIGHTING DIET

The first thing to note is that the more or less acidic flavour of a food is unrelated to its acidifying power. Lemon and vinegar are very acidic tasting but are actually alkalizing! Their acidic flavour results from the presence of organic acids, which, when they come into contact with digestive juices, are converted into very alkalizing mineral salts (notably bicarbonate). In a pain-fighting diet, foods that are acidifying should be limited.

The most acidifying foods are those that contain a lot of sugar, especially when these sugars are refined. So, all sweets and confectionery are very acidifying, as are sugar-laden soft drinks. The same is true, albeit to a lesser extent, of foods containing refined grains (such as white bread, pasta and white rice, especially when precooked). As for industrialized products that combine refined grains and sugar (pastries, biscuits and cakes, for instance), they're high on the list of foods that should be severely limited! Whole grains (such as wholemeal bread and brown rice) pose no such problem; their acidifying potential is virtually neutral.

A second category of foods to limit is meat, especially red meat. Opt instead for poultry or, even better, seafood (fish and shellfish). Like meat, poultry and seafood contain acidifying proteins, but they also provide essential fatty acids (notably omega-3) that attach themselves to inflammatory mechanisms – a kind of internal balance.

To compensate for acidification, turn to vegetables, which contain a lot of alkalizing minerals. Fruits, although sweet, also have an alkalizing effect, although it's less powerful than that of vegetables.

If all this seems a bit complicated, rest assured: the following pages offer a summary of this advice in 8 basic rules.

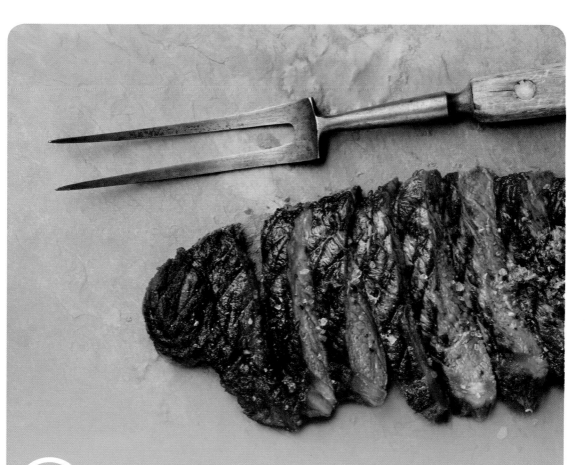

① DECREASE YOUR MEAT CONSUMPTION

Meat (especially red meat) no longer gets a very good press. In recent years, many medical problems have been associated with eating meat. In 2015, the International Agency for Research on Cancer (IARC) officially classified red meat as 'probably carcinogenic to humans'. One thing is certain: excessive consumption of meat, especially red meat, leads to the production of acidic waste that can result in inflammation.

On the other hand, meat contains proteins whose essential components, amino acids, contribute to certain mechanisms involved in a secondary way in dealing with pain. To give just a few examples, isoleucine and leucine amino acids accelerate the healing of damaged tissues; lysine and threonine promote the production of immune cells that protect against infections; and phenylalanine combats the degradation of endorphins, our body-produced painkilling hormones. Try to reduce your meat consumption (to three or four times a week) and focus on light proteins (especially poultry).

② FOCUS ON FISH AND SHELLFISH

Seafood is the best alternative to meat. It provides high-quality proteins, containing all the essential amino acids. Unlike meat, which usually contains saturated fatty acids harmful to your arteries (especially red meat), seafood contains unsaturated fatty acids, which have anti-inflammatory qualities. White fish is much leaner, but its fatty acids are of good quality. Shellfish, meanwhile, is a great source of minerals that combat acidic substances by alkalizing them. So, add seafood to your menus as often as possible.

③ GO LIGHT ON SUGAR!

Avoid refined sugar, such as white sugar, and sugary food like sweets, chocolate spread and fizzy drinks. To sweeten your desserts, opt for less acidifying sugars, such as coconut sugar, agave syrup or even whole cane sugar, which is very rich in alkalizing minerals – go easy on it, though.

'Sugar' isn't just about sweet-flavoured foods. Grains, which, as carbohydrates, break down in our bodies into glucose, are also acidifying when they are refined, such as in white bread, white rice and rusks. And cakes, which combine cereals and refined sugar, are even worse.

We still need valuable carbohydrates, as they are our main source of energy, but in order not to acidify your body, opt for whole grains, such as bread, pasta or rice, which have a negligible impact on internal acidity. And don't forget legumes, such as beans, lentils and chickpeas. Pulses provide an interesting alternative for those who don't like meat or fish, and by combining different ones you'll ensure that your body receives its supply of vegetable proteins.

4 CHOOSE VEGETABLE OILS FOR COOKING AND SEASONING

Although vegetable oils are more or less pH neutral, they do contain antioxidant and anti-inflammatory substances that combat the effects of internal acidification. Note, though, that while some oils are suitable for cooking because their fatty acids support heat, others need to be consumed raw. For cooking, choose olive and rapeseed oils and use other types of oil – such as walnut or sesame – for seasoning. A few types of oil, notably peanut and sunflower, contain pro-inflammatory components and therefore are best avoided.

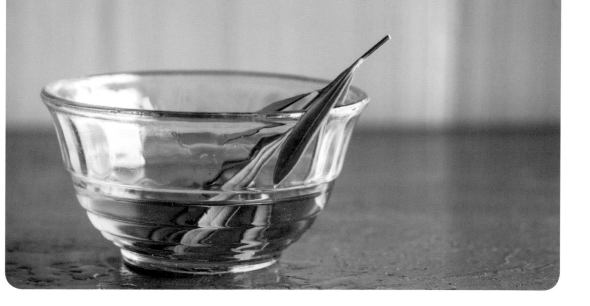

5 BEWARE OF AGED OR HARD CHEESE

Parmesan, for example, is one of the most acidifying foods there is. As a general rule, you're best off choosing fresh cheeses, whose acidifying potential is much lower. You can eat yoghurts for dessert, provided they are sweetened with low-acidifying sugar.

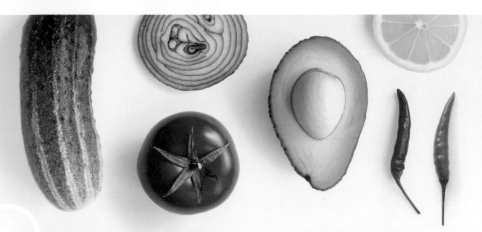

EAT FRESH FRUIT AND VEGETABLES AT EVERY MEAL

Fresh vegetables (or fresh-frozen ones when you're in a hurry) contain a lot of minerals, which compensate for the acidity generated by animal produce and sugars. They also provide antioxidant vitamins and minerals that combat the destructive action of free radicals, and are rich in the fibre that improves digestive transit and maintains intestinal flora. Dietary musts, fruit and vegetables are indispensable every day.

Fresh fruit also provides essential vitamins and minerals. Although fruits are sweet, their acidifying effect is offset by what they provide in terms of nutrients. Aim for two to three servings of fruit per day.

GO EASY ON THE COOKING

Depending on how you cook food, the precious nutrients it contains will be more or less available, easily assimilated and, above all, preserved. Some nutrients, though, such as essential fatty acids and vitamins, are very sensitive to heat. Others resist better but have an unfortunate tendency of becoming lost during the cooking process.

Rather than encouraging an obsessive relationship with food, the aim should be to adopt better habits, with the cooking methods you commonly use playing a part. Learn to avoid nutrient-destroying methods, such as deep-frying, barbecuing or cooking in a very hot oven, in favour of those that release nutrients without damaging them – gentle steaming or cooking in a warm oven, for example. Also avoid cooking vegetables in water, because the minerals have an annoying habit of leaching out into the cooking water. The exception is soup, as you'll be consuming the mineral-loaded cooking water!

⑧ FLAVOUR YOUR DISHES

Herbs and spices delight the palate and can instantly transform a simple dish into a real feast. But their benefits aren't limited purely to their taste; herbs and spices are also truly medicinal. These plant substances form part of the many different cooking traditions worldwide. Europe has long known the virtues of basil, mint, parsley and coriander, while elsewhere in the world, ginger, saffron and turmeric are still used for their health benefits. To alleviate pain, rely on anti-inflammatory herbs and spices.

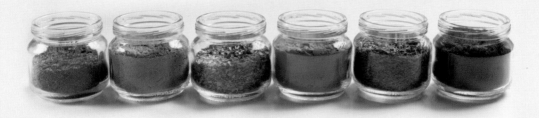

- **Turmeric is the tops!** Numerous studies have shown that turmeric's main active ingredient, curcumin, has a major anti-inflammatory effect. Ayurveda, a medical tradition of ancient India, advocates this spice to combat pain, particularly joint pain. The anti-inflammatory properties of turmeric are even more effective when it's combined with black pepper.
- **Ginger** also has anti-inflammatory and painkilling properties. In 2001, a team of American researchers studied a group of osteoarthritic patients, to whom they gave the equivalent of half a teaspoon of fresh ginger each day. The results were a reduction in joint stiffness and, in particular, less pain – proof that the inflammation of the patients' joint tissues had decreased.
- **Chillies** contain capsaicin, a compound that has been shown in numerous studies to significantly alleviate pain. The most pungent peppers, such as cayenne, are the richest in capsaicin and therefore the most active. Those that contain less capsaicin – Espelette pepper, for example – are therefore less active, although you can put more of this milder pepper in your dishes without burning your palate at the first bite.
- **Thyme and rosemary** also contain various substances that combat tissue inflammation and therefore pain.
- **Many fresh herbs** (such as mint, basil, parsley and coriander) also contain anti-inflammatory compounds, albeit in reduced quantities.

10 FOODS THAT RELIEVE PAIN

Certain foods are particularly active in reducing pain and inflammation. They are mostly, but not exclusively, plant-based foods. Here's a selection that will help you to better manage your pain, provided you consume these foods regularly.

① LEMON
THE ANTACID PAR EXCELLENCE

Not only is lemon a good source of vitamin C (always useful, especially to stimulate tissue healing), but it's also an exceptional antacid. The organic acids it contains turn into alkalizing substances (including bicarbonate) when they make contact with digestive juices.

Lemon juice diluted with water, drunk first thing in the morning for a period of two to three weeks (at each change of season), will greatly benefit your tissues by limiting the acidity that attacks them. As lemon is also slightly diuretic, it promotes the elimination of waste from the kidneys, including the acidic crystals that sometimes lodge in the joints and cause pain.

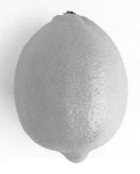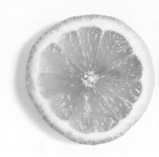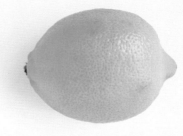

TRY IT!
In addition to using lemon juice as a seasonal cure (see above), you can use it every day in the kitchen.
- **In salad dressings**, instead of vinegar.
- **To add flavour to certain dishes**, such as fish, shellfish, poultry, fried rice, steamed vegetables and fruit salad.

PINEAPPLE
FULL OF NATURAL ANTI-INFLAMMATORY AGENTS

This fruit contains manganese, a trace element that has both antioxidant and anti-inflammatory properties. It also contains bromelain, which combats inflammation by modifying the synthesis of prostaglandins – compounds that are present in many forms in the body. Some of these compounds help to cause inflammation, while others have an anti-inflammatory effect. Bromelain encourages the production of anti-inflammatory prostaglandins. Although bromelain is found mostly in the pineapple's stem and leaves, which are difficult to eat, the flesh still contains quite enough of it to effectively reduce pain.

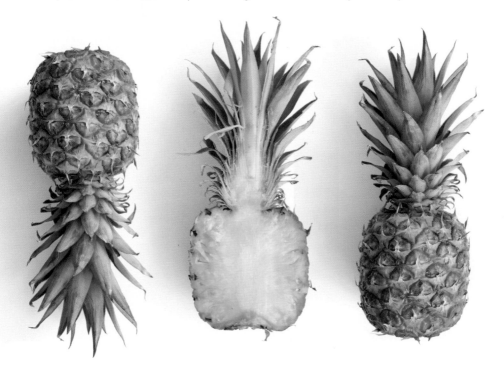

TRY IT!
- **Fresh pineapple can be eaten raw**, as a dessert. You can also use it in pies or fruit salads, and it will pleasantly flavour stewed apples, pears and peaches.
- **You can also add pineapple to sweet-and-savoury dishes**, with chicken breast in a curry, for example.
- **Avoid canned pineapple:** not only is it much sweeter, but it also contains less bromelain.

③ POMEGRANATE
A FAVOURITE PAIN-FIGHTING FOOD

The seeds of this large fruit, which has a hard leather-like skin, contain punicalagin, a compound which decreases inflammation. One study, carried out on mice in 2008, showed clearly that taking them regularly for just ten days reduced pain signals by 70 per cent. And the seeds taste great, too!

TRY IT!
- **When you find ripe pomegranates** (the skin should be very red), enjoy their seeds with a little orange flower water. The combination is delicious, even though it does take quite a while to prepare, as you need to pick out the seeds and take off the whitish pith that lies between them and the skin.
- **The rest of the time, drink organic pomegranate juice** (preferably in the morning), or use it in cooking. Its tangy flavour goes well with poultry and other white meats. But don't cook the juice – add it at the end of cooking, allowing just enough time to heat it through.

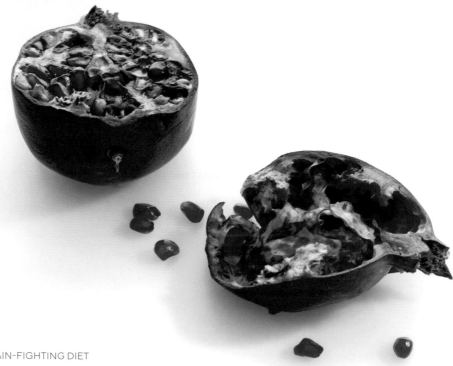

CABBAGE
CALLING A STOP TO INFLAMMATION!

Numerous studies have shown that cabbages and other cruciferous vegetables are good for our health. Some of these veg even have protective properties against various forms of cancer – quite something! All cruciferous vegetables, including green cabbage, red cabbage, broccoli and cauliflower, contain compounds called glucosinolates, which block inflammatory responses. Broccoli deserves a special mention, as it's the richest in sulforaphane, a substance that prevents local inflammation. Many types of pain just can't stand it!

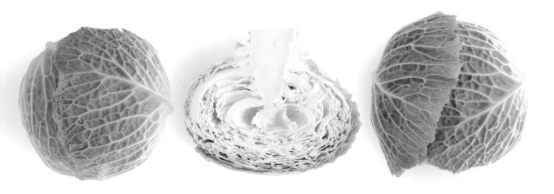

TRY IT!
- **Aim to eat cruciferous vegetables at least two or three times a week.**
- **If you can, eat them raw, in salads:** this is the best way to get your fill of all the beneficial nutrients.
- **If you cook them, favour steaming or braising** as cooking methods, to ensure the vegetables retain most of their essential nutrients.

5 HARICOT BEANS
FULL OF ALKALIZING MINERALS

All legumes (chickpeas, beans, lentils, for example) are excellent foods that provide carbohydrates, vegetable proteins and lots of minerals. Include them regularly in your diet, especially haricot beans, which are particularly rich in potassium, as well as containing calcium, magnesium and iron. Legumes are a good way to neutralize the acidity of meat or fish in the same meal.

TRY IT!
- **If you're in a hurry, use canned white beans** in brine (not cooked). Simply drain, then toss, them with a vinaigrette seasoned with herbs (for example, parsley, basil or coriander) or spices (such as turmeric or cumin). The beans are also very quick to warm through.
- **When you have time, choose dried beans**, which you'll need to soak first for at least 12 hours. Then cook them for about an hour. Season with salt at the end of cooking.
- **The season for fresh beans is short**, but they cook faster than dried beans, are softer and they don't require soaking. So do take advantage of them when they're in season.

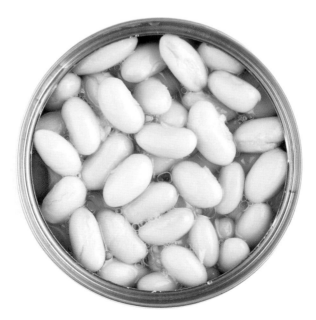

6 OYSTERS
PAINKILLERS FROM THE SEA

This shellfish provides the body with good-quality proteins (and thus painkilling amino acids), anti-inflammatory fatty acids (in small amounts) and, most importantly, a wide range of alkalizing minerals that compensate for oysters' slightly acidifying effect. These minerals include zinc, of which oysters are one of the best sources. Zinc is both antacid and anti-inflammatory, making it a doubly effective painkiller.

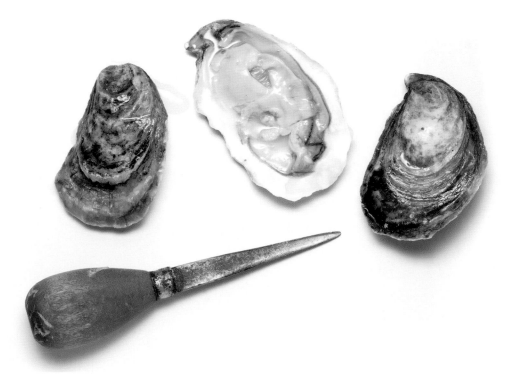

TRY IT!
- **You can, of course, enjoy your oysters raw**, with a drizzle of lemon juice or shallot vinegar and a grinding of pepper. This is the ideal, in terms of nutrition.
- **But don't forget that oysters can also be cooked.** The easiest way to cook them is to cover them in a vegetable-cream sauce, such as coconut, rice or soy, seasoned with herbs or spices, then brown them under the grill for 5 minutes. Simple, fast and delicious!

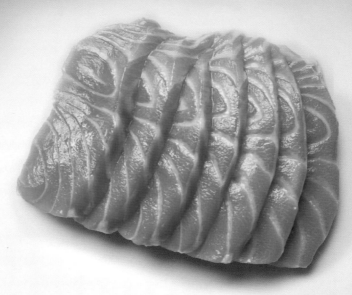

SALMON
FILL UP ON OMEGA-3 ANTI-INFLAMMATORIES

Like sardines, mackerel and anchovies, salmon is a good source of omega-3, which has anti-inflammatory properties. While oily fish are slightly acidifying, the presence of fatty acids such as omega-3 compensates for this harmful effect by blocking pro-inflammatory prostaglandins. Oily fish, especially salmon, also provide many alkalizing minerals. What more could you ask for?

TRY IT!
- **You can eat oily fish often**, because there are endless ways to cook them.
- **Raw, finely chopped with a knife and drizzled with lemon juice**, oily fish make delicious tartare. You can also prepare salmon cut into very thin slices, 'carpaccio' style.
- **Steam cooked**, salmon retains both its flavour and its beneficial nutrients.
- **Think, too, about cooking it 'en papillote'**, or pan-frying it on one side only.
- **Crumble salmon** once cooked, and mix it with pasta or rice. In short, you won't run out of ideas!

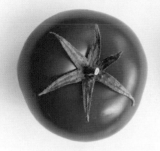
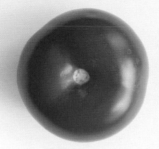
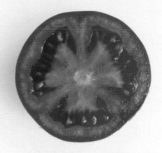

TOMATOES
A REFRESHING PAINKILLER

In 2008, a study conducted by Italian researchers showed the positive effect of regular consumption of tomatoes on rheumatic pain. And it's not surprising, as this common fruit, great in sauces, is packed with anti-inflammatory nutrients and alkalizing minerals. The tomato also provides potassium, which accelerates the elimination of waste from cells. All in all, tomatoes are a great way to provide effective protection against chronic pain, especially during the summer, when they're so refreshing.

TRY IT!
- **Tomatoes are as effective cooked as raw.** Some of the tomato's components, such as lycopene, which is a major antioxidant, gain a great ability for take-up by the body during cooking. Other elements of the tomato, especially its vitamins, are more abundant when the fruit is eaten raw.
- **So here's to tomato sauces**, with onions and herbs, stuffed or Provençal-style tomatoes and tomato salad with feta or mozzarella! The choice is huge.

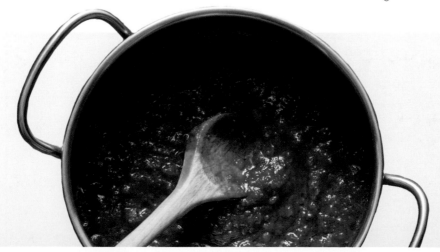

9 BANANAS
ANTACID AND APPETITE-SATISFIER

Potassium, magnesium, calcium, iron – bananas are full of alkalizing minerals, so, despite the sugars they contain, they're not acidifying. Bananas are also an excellent anti-stress food, which is a bonus, because stress intensifies both the perception of pain and the acidification of tissues. As they are very filling, bananas make the perfect snack, instead of sweets.

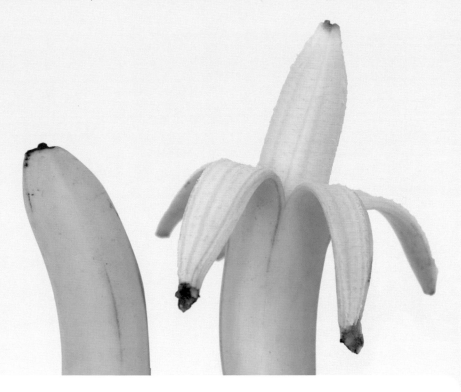

TRY IT!
- **The riper the banana**, the richer it is in sugars. Choose ones that are still firm, with yellow skin and no black spots.
- **Sliced, banana gives consistency** to fruit salads and even to certain sweet-and-savoury starters.
- **As a savoury alternative**, and a change from more usual flavours, puree a banana, season with ginger and anti-inflammatory pepper, and serve alongside white meat or fish.

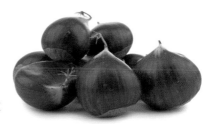

10 CHESTNUTS
MINERAL-PACKED ALKALIZER

For centuries, great chestnut forests have been the pride of the Ardèche and Corsican mountains. These large trees provided carbohydrate-rich fruit that was used instead of cereals, which were rare in those French regions. In fact, chestnuts have an exceptional alkalizing action. They're rich in minerals and trace elements – potassium, phosphorus, magnesium, calcium, iron, manganese, copper and zinc – that combat acidic substances . The time has come to rediscover chestnuts.

TRY IT!
- **You can eat chestnuts plain**, boiled (their thick husk prevents the escape of minerals) or roasted. Score them slightly before cooking, to prevent bursting.
- **Chestnuts make a delicious accompaniment to poultry** – precook them in water, then sauté them in the meat juices. You can use canned chestnuts in brine, too.
- **Chestnut flour is a great (and gluten-free)** alternative to wheat flour for making bread, cakes, pancakes and thick sauces, giving them a very pleasant, subtle flavour.

Making these small changes to your diet will give you a solid nutritional base, especially if you suffer from chronic or recurrent pain. At times when pain is more intense, you can implement other strategies that will provide a faster and lasting result. The rest of the time, your body, rid of excess acidity, will be in better overall shape!

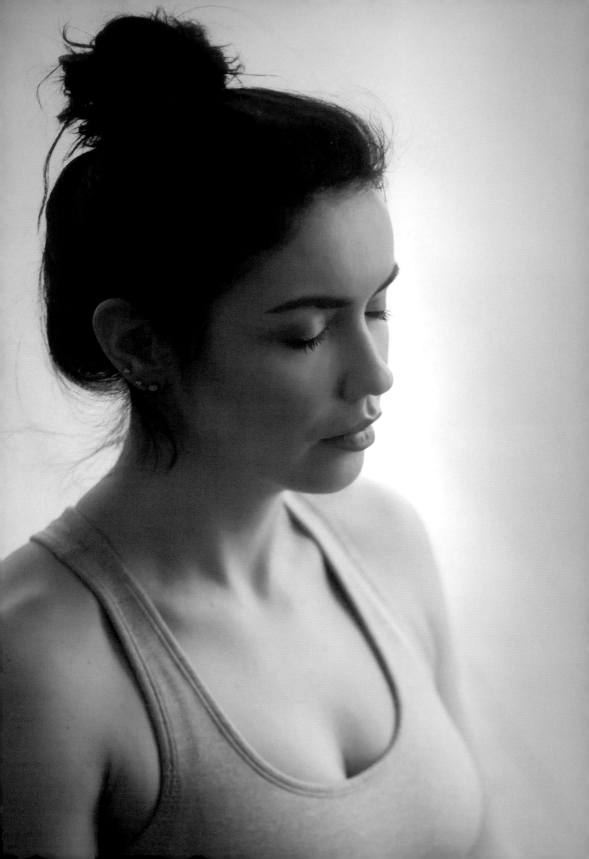

DEEP BREATHING & RELAXATION

This vital chapter rounds up the effects of stress, nervous tension, negative emotions and troubling thoughts on pain management. Remember: it's the nervous system that carries pain signals. To do so, it uses specific fibres, but also particular neurotransmitters. The nervous system is therefore closely involved in manifestations of pain – minor or major, acute or chronic.

2 SIMPLE AND EFFECTIVE WEAPONS AGAINST PAIN

As you'll already have learned, a simple headache can be tormenting or mild depending on whether you're in a stressful, difficult situation or a happy and enjoyable one. The more stressed we are, the more intense the pain feels. Anything that can distract thoughts from pain helps to make it more bearable. Deep-breathing and relaxation exercises, as well as some energizing techniques such as yoga, therefore have their place in the painkilling arsenal.

CALM DOWN, PAIN!

When you're subjected to intense or prolonged stress, your body increases the production of certain neurotransmitters, such as adrenaline, cortisol and acetylcholine. These excite the autonomic nervous system, or more precisely its 'sympathetic' branch. This part of the nervous system manages all our unconscious bodily functions – digestion, sleep, heartbeat and breathing – and is made up of two divisions. The sympathetic (or orthosympathetic) division functions as an accelerator: it stimulates, triggers and activates. The parasympathetic division plays the role of the brake: it calms, slows down and deactivates. The hormonal storm caused by stressful situations pushes the accelerator, to the detriment of the brake. This overstimulation intensifies both inflammation and the sensation of pain.

IMPROVING YOUR PAIN-RESISTANCE THRESHOLD

Each person has a threshold of resistance to pain that is unique to them. Some support pain better than others. Stress, especially when it's frequent or even permanent, erodes pain resistance, which makes these sensations more difficult to bear. Conversely, regular practising of breathing exercises, simple relaxation or yoga postures can help you to cope better with pain and reduce its intensity, which is a useful bonus, especially if you suffer from chronic or recurrent pain.

① BREATHING BETTER TO REDUCE PAIN

Every minute, our lungs absorb and release 6–8 litres (10½–14 pints) of air. We breathe day and night; whether we're awake or asleep, or unconscious as in some types of coma, we're breathing. Breathing is what keeps us alive. Although human beings can survive for several weeks without eating and for a few days without drinking, they can't live for more than a few minutes without breathing. Air is even our first food. Every day, we swallow about 1.5 kg (3¼ lb) of solid food, 2 kg (4½ lb) of liquids and more than 8 kg (17½ lb) of air. It's no wonder, then, that breathing is fundamental to our equilibrium and health.

Breathing is absorbing the oxygen that's essential to cell life and expelling carbon dioxide. And the good news is that carbon dioxide, the gaseous residue of cellular metabolism, is very acidifying, so the better we eliminate it, the better we protect the body from excess acidity.

This physiological dimension aside, breathing is like a thread stretched between your conscious will and your unconscious biological life. It's the only one of your bodily functions that you can modulate at will just by thinking about it. Try it now: without putting down this book, try holding your breath for a few seconds, then speed up your breathing, then slow it down. You can probably do this easily. Try to do the same with your heartbeat: it's impossible! However, by controlling your breathing, you can also modify your heart rate.

This is of great help in managing stress and emotions. By changing the pace of your breathing to make it slower, deeper and more regular, you will rebalance your autonomic nervous system and modify the production of neurotransmitters – two valuable assets in neutralizing pain.

THE MOVEMENTS OF THE CHEST DURING BREATHING

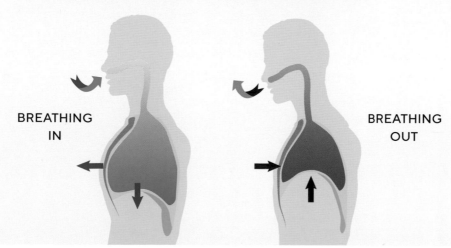

BREATHING IN

BREATHING OUT

Finally, breathing exercises have a calming effect at the psycho-emotional level. It's no coincidence that all relaxation and meditation techniques, as well as most mind–body approaches, such as yoga, qigong, mindfulness meditation, therapeutic hypnosis and sophrology, focus primarily on regulation of breathing. This is explained by the fact that, beyond calming you physically, slowing down your breathing acts as a psychological sedative. Just focusing on your breathing will help to divert your attention from obsessive negative thoughts. This simple action is enough to reduce emotional attacks and even keep them at bay.

Breathing exercises establish a state of mental relaxation that becomes automatic over time when you practise them regularly. After a few weeks, the secretion of neurohormones will level out naturally, favouring calm- and pleasure-inducing ones (mainly dopamine and serotonin) at the expense of those released in response to stress and nervous tension (adrenaline and cortisol). Notably, your pain–perception threshold will gradually change.

To learn how to breathe better will take you, initially, only 5 minutes, three times a day. You can practise at any time and set a breathing–exercise timetable to suit you. However, the ideal is to practise 5 minutes of deep and conscious breathing in the morning, just after waking up (so that you begin your day in peace) and again in the evening when you go to bed (so that you start the night relatively stress free). You can plan the additional exercise time to suit you. Also, if your pain is intense, you can do these exercises more often or for longer.

TRY IT!
- **To start with, you'll need to isolate yourself** somewhere calm to practise. Close your eyes and find a comfortable position.
- **During the day**, it's best to do these exercises sitting rather than lying down, so you don't fall asleep.
- **In the evening**, you can do your exercises lying on your bed. If you fall asleep before you've finished, so much the better!
- **Gradually, as you get into the habit**, you'll be able to breathe in this way anywhere – on public transport, in a meeting, during a difficult family discussion or even standing in the middle of a crowd – as soon as you feel the need, without anyone around you noticing.
- **These few minutes a day** will gradually register in your subconscious and you'll breathe differently even when you're not thinking about it.

BREATHING TO LOWER STRESS LEVELS

This breathing technique has its roots in applied neuroscience. Short though it is, it will enable you to quickly reduce your level of nervous tension. Alternating the breathing between right and left nostrils provides information directly to the brain, which reacts by instilling a feeling of calm. This form of breathing inhibits areas of stress and activates those of pleasure and positive emotions. It thus prevents (or alleviates) the imbalance between the two divisions of the autonomic nervous system (sympathetic and parasympathetic) and stimulates the production of serotonin, the neurohormone related to relaxation and calm.

Taking only about 5 minutes, the exercise can be repeated several times a day, whenever you feel the need.

TRY IT!

- **Sit on the edge of a chair**, keeping your back straight. Your feet should be on the floor, your hands flat on your thighs. Relax your shoulders.
- **Start by taking a deep breath**, then expel a deep sigh with your mouth open.
- **Cover your left nostril with your left thumb**, then inhale through your right nostril while you slowly count to three.
- **Exhale in the same way**, but pursing your lips (as though you wanted to prevent the air escaping) and tightening your abdominal muscles, while you count to six. Repeat three times.
- **Release your left nostril and cover your right nostril with your middle finger** (without changing hands). Inhale through your left nostril, counting slowly to three.
- **Release your right nostril and cover the left again** with your thumb to breathe out, while counting to six. Repeat three times.
- **Continue in this way, alternating the two nostrils**, for about 5 minutes before resuming your normal breathing.

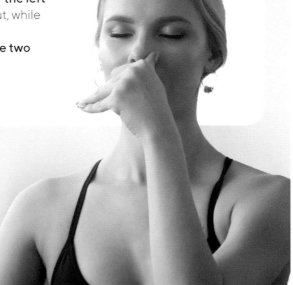

BREATHING TO NEUTRALIZE TEMPORARY PAIN

As soon as you feel pain coming on, take 2 or 3 minutes to neutralize it. This exercise is particularly effective in fighting joint pain that manifests itself in sudden bursts, provided you practise it as soon as the pain appears.

TRY IT!

- **Wherever you are, sit on the edge of a chair**, keeping your back straight. Your feet should be on the floor, your hands flat on your thighs and your shoulders relaxed.
- **Close your eyes** or, if you're not alone, try to keep your eyes fixed on some vague point to help you stay focused on what's happening inside you.
- **Inhale calmly**, while counting slowly to three or four, then exhale, counting to six or eight. Adapt these durations to your usual breathing rhythms, but focus on keeping the exhalation twice as long as the inhalation.
- **Try to stay focused on your breathing**, feeling the air skimming your nostrils as it enters and leaves your body.
- **Continue the exercise** for at least 3 minutes, then slowly return to your normal breathing and open your eyes again.
- **Practise this exercise** whenever you feel pain rising. Focusing on your breathing will distract you from the pain.

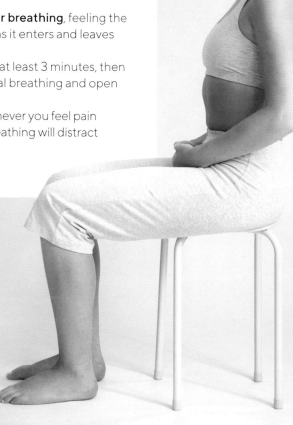

BREATHING TO CALM CHRONIC PAIN

This type of breathing is also inspired by neuroscientific research. It will enable you to create, gradually, an 'interior space' that pain can't penetrate – a 'pain-free' space. Each time you practise this exercise, this space will become stronger and you'll be able to access it more and more easily. You'll be able to 'crack' the pain, just as you 'cracked' stress in the first exercise.

TRY IT!

- **Sit in the same position** as for previous exercises (see opposite), then take a deep breath and, with your mouth open, exhale in a big sigh.
- **Inhale slowly while counting to three**, then hold your breath for the same length of time.
- **Exhale more slowly, counting to six.** Contract your abs to expel the air from your lungs.
- **Relax your stomach muscles, without inhaling**, while you count to three. Relax your face and shoulders, too.
- **At this point, your brain will be waiting for you to breathe in.** This is a vital issue for your brain, so it goes into 'survival mode', disconnecting not only negative thoughts but also the nerve loops that transmit pain, and thus creating an inner 'bubble' of mental and neuromuscular peace.
- **After 3 seconds, inhale again** and resume the breathing cycle in the same way.
- **Practise this breathing technique** for 10 minutes, repeating it at least three times a day. By repeating this exercise, you'll gradually stretch this 'peace bubble' and anchor it deep in your brain.

RELAXATION FOR BETTER PAIN RESISTANCE

We can't escape stress. And that's good, because it's an exceptional source of stimulation. Without the stress of their dangerous and uncomfortable daily lives, our distant ancestors wouldn't have sought to improve their conditions. It's stress that, over thousands of years, has pushed us to act, create and invent. The problem, therefore, isn't stress itself, but rather the badly managed accumulation of stress, which ultimately unbalances our nervous system and, as a consequence, intensifies painful phenomena.

By learning how to better manage potentially stressful situations, you'll be having an effect on many levels simultaneously. First, you'll be freeing your mind and emotions from nervous tension and obsessive thoughts. Next, you'll quickly feel your body ridding itself of accumulated tension, such as muscular tension and joint pain. Meanwhile, behind the scenes, balance will be being restored gradually to all your bodily functions. Finally, this sweep of beneficial effects will culminate in a long-lasting benefit: by regularly practising a relaxation method, you'll improve your resistance threshold to stress and pain. As they're gradually freed up, your body, mind and emotions will regain their ability to manage the troubling situations of everyday life, which will help you to cope better with pain when it does appear.

There are numerous relaxation methods you can draw on to find practical exercises to suit you, including sophrology, progressive muscle relaxation (Jacobson's technique) and Schultz's autogenic training. All offer exercises that combine work on the breath (breathing), the body (physical relaxation) and psychological tension. Most of these techniques also include work involving mental images (visualizations).

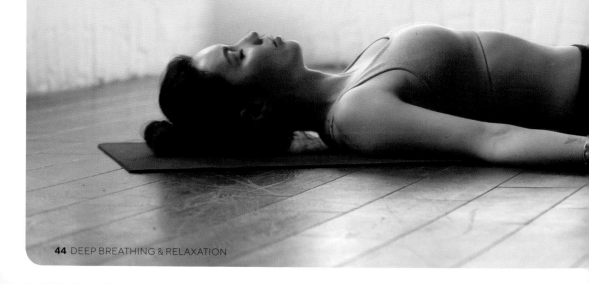

If the time seems right to you to master one of these well-established techniques, seize the moment and give it a go! If you don't feel the urge, nor have the energy to embark on such an adventure right now, simply practise at least one of the exercises below every day. You can take your pick, depending on the time you have available and the immediate results you're hoping to achieve. The rapid improvement you'll feel will perhaps give you the motivation you need to explore a more traditional relaxation technique in more depth.

TRY IT!
- **These exercises are mostly done** lying down.
- **During the daytime**, lie on a mat, or directly on the floor if it's not too firm for you. If necessary, put a small cushion under your neck for support.
- **In the evening**, lie down on your bed – but don't wait until you're really sleepy, or you'll drop off before the end of the exercise session!
- **You can do these breathing exercises with music, if you wish.** Choose some gentle (classical or relaxing) music, or sound recordings from nature, such as waves, birdsong or rain. Pick a piece of a duration that matches your exercise. It will then serve as both a relaxation aid and a stopwatch.

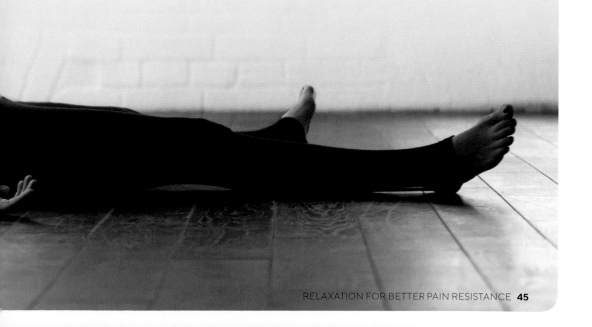

A BASIC EXERCISE TO RELIEVE CHRONIC PAIN

If your pain is permanent, or at least regular, you can practise this exercise every night before falling asleep. If you incorporate it into your daily life, it will also help to soothe your stress levels and improve your sleep.

TRY IT!
- **Do the exercise lying on your back on your bed**, before you fall asleep. Put your head flat on the mattress, or on a thin pillow – your neck should remain aligned with your spine. Close your eyes.
- **Start by adopting a deep and regular breathing pattern** – the expiration should always be longer than the inhalation. The easiest way to achieve this is to focus your attention on the expiration.
- **Contract your abdominal muscles** to slow down your exhalation, and keep breathing out until your lungs are completely empty. Then breathe in naturally, without thinking about it.
- **Breathe like this for a few minutes, then imagine a soothing stream of golden light** entering your body at the top of your head and spreading throughout your body.
- **Direct this light** to the place of your pain: your head, joints, belly or wherever.
- **When you inhale, imagine the light bathing this painful area**, like a regenerative liquid. When you exhale, imagine the light carrying the pain, inflammation and toxins away with it, evacuating them through the soles of your feet.
- **Continue this breathing and visualization as you fall asleep** – for at least 10 minutes.
- **If you practise this exercise regularly**, it will provide you with long–term pain relief.

A PAINKILLING VISUALIZATION

This exercise is inspired by a technique called cardiac coherence. The technique aims to recreate coherence between the electromagnetic signals emitted by the neurons in your heart and those in your cranial cavity – for your heart, too, has a very active and powerful neural network. When the heart and brain act together, all your metabolic functioning improves. In addition, in these moments of perfect coherence, your mind receives all the signals you're sending it 'loud and clear', including signals that soothe tension and, above all, pain.

TRY IT!
- **Sit in the same position** as for the breathing exercises. (Once you've become accustomed to these exercises, you can also practise them lying down, without the risk of immediately falling asleep.)
- **Start by breathing calmly and deeply**, eyes closed, without straining and without counting, until you begin to feel relaxed.
- **Then, without changing the rhythm of your breathing**, focus your attention on your heart. Feel it beating. Imagine that the air is entering and leaving your body not through your nose but through your heart itself, as if it had a small mouthlike orifice.
- **Keep breathing until you feel a sort of heat or expansion in your chest.** At this point, the neurons in your cranial cavity have become coherent with your cardiac neurons.
- **Take advantage of this state of coherence** to send soothing signals to your heart and brain. The coherence that has developed between the two 'opens the door' to mental signals, which will make your body react in a way that alleviates your pain.
- **For example, say to yourself,** 'I feel my pain ebbing; it's fading, then disappearing.' Or say, 'My body is increasing its production of endorphins to rid itself of pain.'
- **Find a formula that suits you and with which you feel comfortable**, then continue the exercise by repeating the phrases above for at least 10 minutes. Continued repetition is necessary at the beginning in order to create a kind of reflex between your heart and your brain.
- **You can repeat this exercise several times a day** at times when you have a lot of pain. It will take effect more and more quickly.
- **Once your heart and brain have become accustomed to the exercise,** 2 or 3 minutes will be enough for it to take effect.

AN EXERCISE TO LOWER YOUR STRESS AND PAIN THRESHOLD

Here's an exercise that's also based on applied neuroscience. Studies have shown that the simple act of smiling activates the same parts of your brain as when you are truly feeling happy. So smile away – especially as this 'joy activation' will cause your brain to secrete anti-stress hormones (notably serotonin) and painkilling hormones (such as endorphins). You'll win on all fronts!

TRY IT!

- **You can practise this exercise in any position**, as long as you can close your eyes for a few minutes.
- **Take a few calm, deep breaths, then imagine yourself smiling.** You can actually smile, as well (even if you don't really feel like it right now!).
- **Imagine the energy of this smile going back into your cranial cavity** and bathing your brain, producing a feeling of total wellbeing.
- **Then imagine the smile descending through every part of your body:** down into your neck, shoulders, arms, hands, chest, stomach, hips, legs and feet.
- **When the smile arrives in a painful area**, stay there for a few moments.
- **This exercise takes effect quickly.** In all, it should take you less than a minute.
- **Return to your normal state of consciousness and open your eyes.** Try to hold on to the joyful feeling that has swept through you for as long as possible. And the next time you feel overwhelmed by stress or pain, begin again!

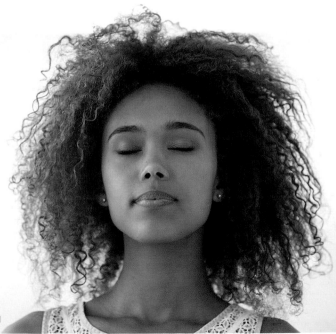

A RELAXATION EXERCISE TO COMBAT MUSCULAR PAIN

This exercise will help to relax your whole body, which can carry much mental and emotional tension. All those muscular, postural and joint pains will subside and eventually disappear, and in the process you'll also relax your nerves, which will protect you against further painful contractions.

TRY IT!
- **You can perform this relaxation** during the day, or in the evening at bedtime – but be careful not to fall asleep before you reach the end!
- **Close your eyes** and start breathing calmly and deeply, but without straining.
- **Keeping the same breathing rhythm**, contract your calf muscles (right and left). Focus your attention on what you're feeling.
- **Then release the tension** you've become aware of.
- **Continue in the same way**, contracting then relaxing the muscles in your thighs, then in your buttocks, stomach, arms, shoulders, neck and, finally, face.
- **For this exercise to be effective**, you must really feel what your body is telling you when you contract your muscles. It's as you become conscious of where you're tensing up that you'll be able to release this tension effectively.
- **When you have time**, do the whole exercise.
- **When you need to calm down during the day**, practise it sitting down (see the position on page 42) and focus only on your arms and shoulders, your thighs and calves, or wherever else you feel uncomfortably tense.

Now that you've familiarized yourself with some general painkilling techniques – diet, breathing and stress management – the time has come to add more specific treatments, adapted to specific types of pain.

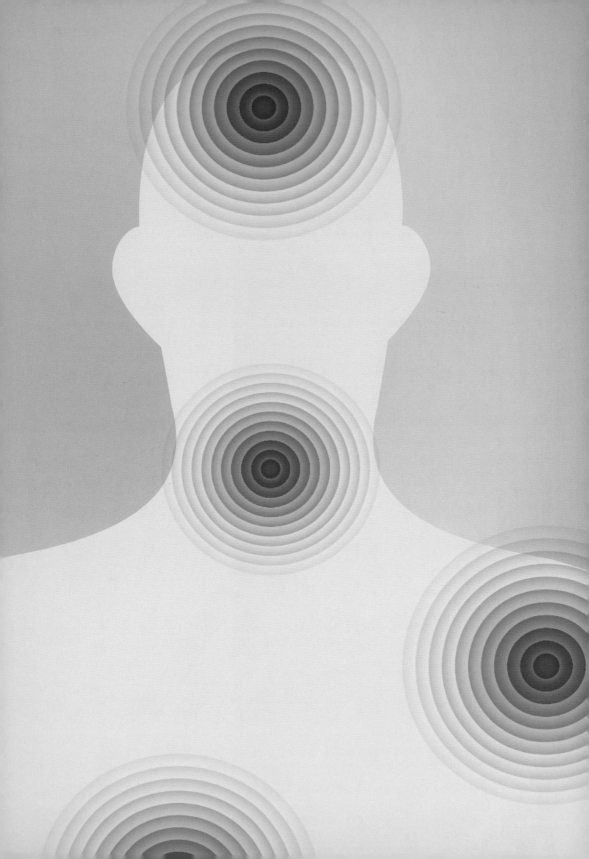

4

PRACTICAL ADVICE FOR COMMON AILMENTS

As well as applying the general advice given in earlier chapters, you can choose from specific pain-management treatments depending on where in your body the pain is localized, where it originated and so on. Different types of pain respond to different types of treatments, based on natural products or traditional remedies. Whether you're suffering from migraine or toothache, joint pain or stomach ache, bruising or burning, you'll find something here to relieve your pain, or even make it disappear for good.

NATURAL REMEDIES FOR 10 COMMON AILMENTS

1 HEADACHES

Cephalalgia is the medical term for all types of headache, including migraine (pain in half of the skull), ophthalmic headache (related to eyestrain) and headaches of neural, hormonal or digestive origin. In all cases, headaches, which can vary in intensity, are distressing because it's very difficult to think and concentrate when your head feels like it's trapped in a vice.

Women are more affected than men by headaches, whether occasionally or frequently. A person is deemed to suffer from chronic headaches when they've experienced at least five seizures in the previous twelve months, each lasting at least 48 hours. If you frequently get headaches, seek medical advice to determine their origin. You'll then be better equipped to treat the source of the problem. In addition, you can administer the following treatments whenever you suffer from a headache. The sooner you act, the more effective they will be.

A FEVERFEW INFUSION

The feverfew plant, also sometimes called bachelor's buttons, has been used since ancient times to soothe pain, particularly headaches. Its efficacy for this traditional use has been scientifically proven. Some scientific studies suggest that feverfew may reduce the frequency and severity of migraine headaches.

TRY IT!
- **Add 1 level tablespoon of dried feverfew** to a large cup of boiling water. Leave to infuse for 5 minutes, then filter and drink.
- **If your headache is isolated**, drink two or three cups a day.
- **If the headache is recurrent**, continue the treatment for a week: drink a large cup as soon as you feel a headache coming on, and continue to drink two large cups a day for the rest of the week.

A MASSAGE WITH PEPPERMINT ESSENTIAL OIL

When distilled, peppermint, an ancient medicinal plant, yields an essential oil that has decongestant, anti-inflammatory and antispasmodic properties. Most importantly, it's a great painkiller and provides rapid relief – good news if you suffer from headaches.

TRY IT!
- **If the headache is quite localized**, put a drop of peppermint essential oil on the tips of both your index fingers, then rub the spot where your headache is – for example, your forehead (be careful to avoid touching your eyes), temples or neck. Repeat an hour later if the pain persists.
- **If the headache is more widespread and diffuse**, soak a compress in cold water, then add 2 or 3 drops of peppermint essential oil to it. Lie down in a quiet place and put the compress high on your forehead. Leave it to work for at least 10 minutes.

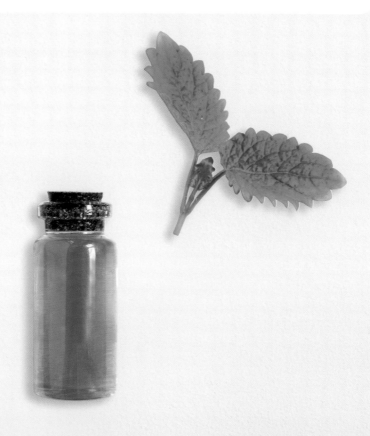

A MEADOWSWEET POULTICE

A traditional medicinal plant, meadowsweet has many virtues, including anti-inflammatory and antispasmodic properties, which make it particularly valuable for those who suffer from headaches. Meadowsweet played its part in the story of the famous aspirin. It was from substances contained in its beautiful white flowers, combined with others present in willow bark, that chemists synthesized the drug at the end of the nineteenth century. It's no wonder, then, that this plant is a good ally when you're suffering from a headache.

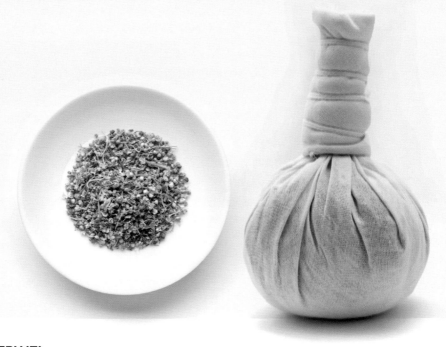

TRY IT!
- **When meadowsweet is used in a poultice, its beneficial constituents** act through the skin.
- **Put 5 tablespoons** of dried meadowsweet into a bowl, then pour over a little boiling water to cover. Mix well and leave to infuse for 15 minutes. Filter to separate the plant material from the concentrated infusion.
- **Soak a compress in the infusion and spread the leaves on top.** Carefully place this on your forehead or neck (wherever you feel pain), with the plant material against your skin. Keep it in place for 15–20 minutes, preferably while lying in a dark, quiet place. If the headache persists, repeat up to twice a day.
- **You can also** consume meadowsweet in an infusion. Add a level tablespoonful of dried meadowsweet to a large cup of boiling water, then leave to infuse for 8 minutes before filtering. Drink two cups a day.

A POINT TO STIMULATE ON THE HAND

This point, according to Chinese medicine, is on the meridian, or energy channel, of the large intestine. So, what is its relationship to headaches? The meridian begins at the tip of the index finger and goes up the arm, then from the shoulder and neck to the skull. An energy blockage along this pathway can cause headaches. To relieve the blockage, just massage a specific point. It's also a useful anti-stress point when the headache is linked to nervous tension.

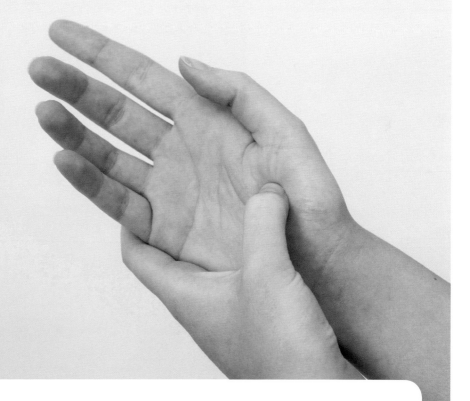

TRY IT!
- **Start by rubbing your palms together**, then interlace your fingers as though you're washing your hands.
- **Once your hands are warmed up**, place your left thumb on the fleshy part of your right hand between the thumb and forefinger.
- **Look for the point** located at the bottom of the 'fork' between thumb and forefinger, next to the joint, and press. This point is usually a little painful.
- **Massage lightly** in a clockwise direction, then in the opposite direction.
- **Continue for 2–3 minutes.** Do the same with the other hand. Repeat several times a day.

② ORAL PAIN

There are many reasons why the mouth may become painful, including dental cavities, infections, inflammation of the gums and mouth ulcers. These aren't serious conditions (unless they're left untreated), but they can produce troubling discomfort and even intense pain. If you have severe toothache, you'll need to pay a visit to the dentist. But there's nothing to stop you doing something to alleviate the pain while you're waiting for your appointment. Other types of mouth-related pain can be managed by improving your dental and oral hygiene and by adopting certain effective natural remedies.

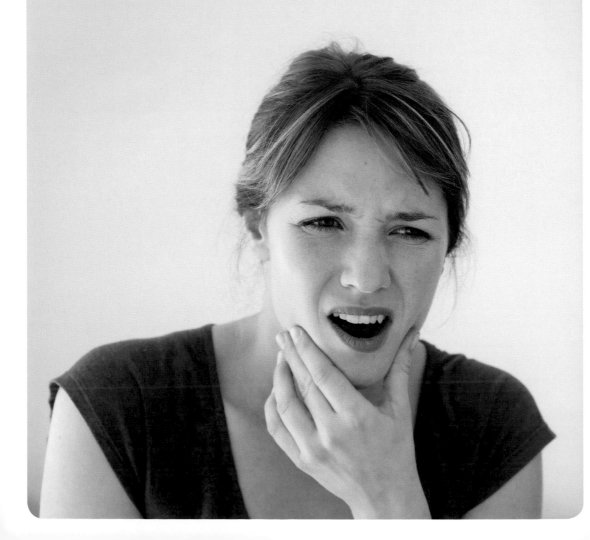

MOUTH ULCERS

A mouth ulcer is a small, superficial and most often isolated ulceration of the mucous membrane of the oral cavity (gums, tongue or inner cheeks). It usually has a yellowish centre ringed with red. When mouth ulcers reappear frequently, the condition is called aphthous stomatitis. An ulcer is painful to the touch, and the slightest movement of the mouth or tongue can cause an unpleasant, burning sensation, which can make it difficult to even eat or talk. Untreated, common mouth ulcers will heal themselves in ten to fifteen days and leave no trace, but why suffer so long when a few simple remedies can relieve the pain?

A PLUM JUICE MOUTHWASH

Plums are exceptionally rich in copper, a trace element that stimulates immune defences. Some mouth ulcers are caused by an infection, but even if this isn't the case, better oral protection routines will help to make them disappear faster.

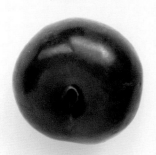 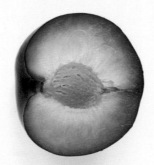 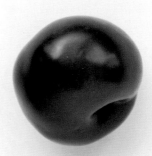

TRY IT!
- Put two or three large fresh plums into a juicer.
- Dilute this juice with an equal volume of mineral water and use as a mouthwash.
- Take time to really bathe the mouth ulcers.
- Leave the diluted juice in your mouth for 15 minutes, then rinse your mouth thoroughly with clear water to remove the sugar from the fruit.
- Repeat morning and evening.

A LEMON JUICE MOUTHWASH

Lemon juice is antacid, cleansing, antibacterial and healing. In other words, it's the perfect remedy for beating mouth ulcers once and for all, and for dealing with the pain they can cause.

TRY IT!

- **Squeeze half a lemon**, preferably organic, carefully filtering the juice through a fine strainer or piece of muslin.
- **Dip a cotton bud** in the juice, then generously coat any mouth ulcers with it.
- **Dilute the remainder of the lemon juice** with a little mineral water and make a mouthwash to complete the treatment.
- **Repeat** several times a day.

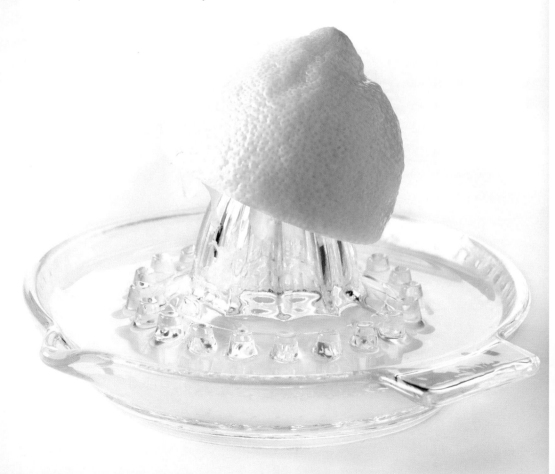

FRESH BASIL LEAVES

A culinary herb, basil also has many beneficial properties that help to fight mouth ulcers. Basil improves digestion (some mouth ulcers have digestive causes), is calming (sometimes the cause is stress related) and contains antiseptic substances. All of this makes basil highly effective, whatever the cause of your mouth ulcers.

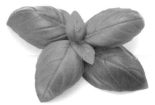

TRY IT!

- **Pick some leaves** from a large-leaved, preferably organic, basil plant. Rinse them thoroughly.
- **Chew the leaves for a long time**, as though you were chewing gum. The idea is not to swallow them, but to work them between your teeth in order to extract all the juice.
- **Repeat** several times a day.
- **If you don't like the taste of basil**, you can use flat-leaf parsley instead. It's less effective, but better than nothing!

BAY LEAF ESSENTIAL OIL

It would be difficult to find a more effective remedy to deal with all the unwanted germs – bacteria, viruses or fungi – that colonize the mouth and disrupt precious oral micro-organisms. In addition, this essential oil has painkilling and healing properties – a winning cocktail!

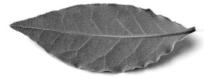

TRY IT!

- **Nothing's easier:** simply pour a drop of bay leaf essential oil on the end of your little finger, then place it directly on the mouth ulcer.
- **Massage it in lightly.**
- **Repeat** three times a day.

GINGIVITIS

This is an inflammation of the gums, the pink flesh that surrounds both the root of the teeth and the jawbone in which they're inserted. When inflamed, the gums become red, swollen and painful; they bleed at the slightest touch (with a toothbrush, for example) and become sensitive to the cold. In itself, gingivitis isn't a serious condition, but if left untreated it can weaken the supporting tissues of the tooth and evolve into the gum disease periodontitis. That's why it's best to act without delay.

A PEPPERMINT AND BICARBONATE OF SODA (BAKING SODA) MOUTHWASH

Gingivitis can be caused, or made worse, by too much acidity in the oral environment. Bicarbonate of soda (baking soda) is an antacid, and peppermint is antibacterial, refreshing and, most importantly, pain relieving. A treatment combining bicarbonate of soda (baking soda) and peppermint essential oil is therefore extremely effective in relieving the discomfort caused by gingivitis.

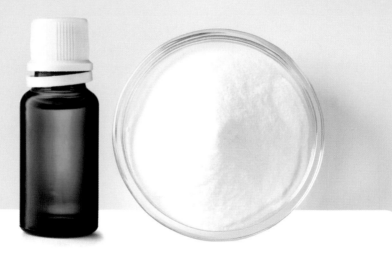

TRY IT!
- **Put 2 teaspoons of bicarbonate of soda (baking soda)** in a glass and add 2 drops of peppermint essential oil.
- **Stir** so that the powder absorbs the essential oil, then half fill the glass with water (at room temperature). Stir again.
- **Use as a mouthwash**, morning and evening (and at midday, too, if you wish), until the pain and bleeding subside.

A VINEGAR RINSE

Vinegar is another very alkalizing natural product – helpful for balancing your oral environment, which is probably too acidic. This rinse is an extremely simple and highly effective treatment, as vinegar is also antibacterial and able to relieve pain a little.

TRY IT!
- **Pour 2 tablespoons of organic cider vinegar** into half a glass of warm (or room-temperature) water. Stir well.
- **After you've thoroughly cleaned your teeth** (using a soft brush to protect your gums), rinse your mouth with the vinegar water.
- **Bathe your mouth well**, to ensure that your gums are sufficiently in contact with the vinegar.
- **Repeat morning and evening** until the unpleasant symptoms subside.

A HAND MASSAGE TO STIMULATE DENTAL ENERGY

Our hands carry 'reflex zones' that correspond to various parts of the body, including the teeth and gums. According to Chinese energy medicine, by massaging your hands regularly, you'll stimulate the energy that 'feeds' these tissues – another weapon in your arsenal to fight against gum pain.

TRY IT!
- **The zone corresponding to the gums** is found on each thumb, just below the root of the nail.
- **The zones corresponding to the teeth** are located on the other fingers, also just below the nails.
- **Prepare a massage oil** by adding 3 drops of tea tree essential oil to a teaspoon of wheatgerm or jojoba oil. Mix well.
- **Use this mixture to first massage your whole hands:** palms, backs of the hands and fingers.
- **Next, focus on the zones corresponding to the gums and teeth.** Massage each finger for 1 minute, especially if the area is painful.
- **Finish by rubbing your hands together.**
- **Do this massage** at least once a day – twice, if possible.

TOOTHACHE

Decay, gnawing away at the dentine and touching the nerve cavity, is most often the cause of toothache. Sometimes an infection sets in, which increases the pain. You'll need to visit the dentist – but, before you go, you can ease the pain with these simple routines.

A THYME MOUTHWASH

Thyme is packed with antiseptic substances. Used as a mouthwash, it will cleanse your oral cavity and eliminate germs. In addition, it has an anti-inflammatory effect, which means it's a welcome pain reliever when you're suffering from toothache.

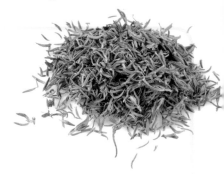

TRY IT!
- **Boil** enough water to fill a small glass.
- **When the water comes to the boil**, remove from the heat and add 1 tablespoon of dried thyme.
- **Leave to infuse** for 10 minutes, then filter well.
- **Use as a mouthwash**, taking good care to bathe the painful tooth.
- **Repeat** at least twice a day.

A CLOVE IN THE TOOTH

It's no coincidence that the smell of cloves immediately evokes the dentist's surgery. This spice contains active ingredients that are cleansing, disinfecting and, especially, pain relieving. Cloves will help to stem the pain while you wait for more targeted dental care.

TRY IT!
- **If you have a big hole in your tooth** (when you lose a filling, for example), use a whole clove. Detach the little ball from its stem, slip it into the tooth and leave it to do its job quietly.
- **If the hole isn't large enough to fit a whole clove**, try some ground cloves. Using the tip of your finger, place some of the powder in the dental cavity and leave it to work. Repeat every 2 hours.

A MASSAGE WITH CLOVE ESSENTIAL OIL

The essential oil extracted from cloves concentrates all its active ingredients. It helps to relieve toothache when the tooth doesn't appear damaged, which could mean either the decay is developing inside the tooth or the pain is due to inflammation of the root. But be warned: the oil has a very pungent taste. If you really don't like cloves, abstain!

TRY IT!
- **Put a drop** (only one!) of clove essential oil on the tip of your index finger.
- **Massage the gum** around the painful tooth, outside and inside.
- **Repeat** as often as necessary.

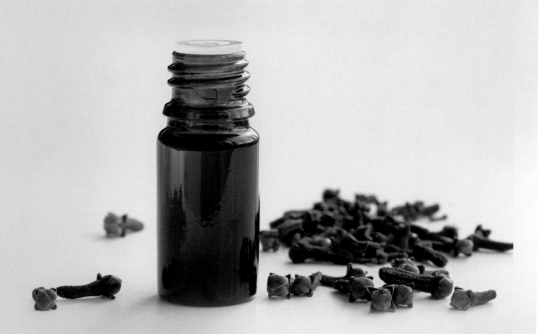

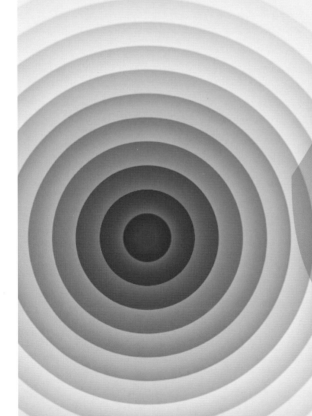

③EAR, NOSE AND THROAT PAIN

The zone that consists of the ears, nose and throat is vulnerable to irritation, inflammation and infections, which can sometimes be very painful. These organs are interconnected, so it's best to deal with them together. When problems are accompanied by a fever (even a slight rise in temperature), you should see a doctor to ensure that you treat the underlying infection. In any case, whether or not you're prescribed medical treatment, certain simple natural remedies can help you to neutralize the pain.

SORE THROAT

If you open your mouth to check the base of your throat in a mirror when you have a sore throat, you'll notice that it's red and possibly also shiny and swollen. You may also have trouble swallowing, which can be very painful. A sore throat could be the result of either a simple irritation or an infection that shouldn't be taken lightly (watch out, particularly, if you're running a fever). In either case, there are localized treatments that will calm the tissues and relieve pain.

HOMEOPATHIC GRANULES

It's not always easy to treat yourself with homeopathic remedies – the choice is often complex, as symptoms can be many and varied. This isn't the case, though, with a sore throat, even if you have full-blown tonsillitis. Just look at your throat and choose the product based on its appearance. If you don't see results after 48 hours, you've not chosen the right remedy and should see a doctor, especially if you have a fever. You can buy homeopathic granules from health food shops or online suppliers.

TRY IT!

- **If your throat is red and shiny**, take 3 granules of Mercurius solubilis 9C and 3 granules of Belladonna 5C (at the same time) four times a day.
- **If your throat is pink and swollen**, take 3 granules of Apis 5C four times a day.
- **If your throat is very dark red**, take 3 granules of Phytolacca 5C four times a day.
- **If your throat is covered with small white dots**, take 3 granules of Mercurius solubilis 5C four times a day.
- **If the pain and inflammation affect only the left side of the throat**, take 3 granules of Lachesis 5C four times a day.
- **If the pain and inflammation affect only the right side of the throat**, take 3 granules of Lycopodium 5C four times a day.
- **While waiting** for the treatment to take effect, you can also use any of the localized treatments that follow.

A PROPOLIS REMEDY

As well as honey, bees make propolis, a kind of paste that they use to disinfect the hive and make it watertight. Another gift to us humans, propolis is rich in antibiotic compounds and natural essences. It's particularly useful in winter, as it quickly relieves sore throats and prevents their reappearance.

TRY IT!
- **Natural propolis**, which comes in small pieces of 1–2 g, can be bought online.
- **Chew a piece** slowly, as if you were chewing gum. Keep it in your mouth as long as possible (at least 15 minutes).
- **Repeat** two or three times a day. Continue for two to three weeks after the sore throat has stopped, and you'll be free all winter.
- **If you don't like the taste of propolis** (it's quite strong), choose a propolis product instead – for example, a spray to cleanse the throat or lozenges to suck.

A PHYTOLACCA GARGLE

Phytolacca (pokeweed) is a shrubby plant that's rarely used in herbal medicine but very common in homeopathy. Here, you'll use the mother tincture (a maceration with alcohol). This mixture is normally used to steep homeopathic granules, but you're going to use it to relieve the pain in your throat.

TRY IT!
- **Phytolacca mother tincture** can be bought online from suppliers of homeopathic remedies.
- **Pour 30 drops** into half a glass of warm water and mix.
- **Use this liquid** as a gargle. Bathe the base of your throat in the liquid for as long as you can, but don't swallow it.
- **Repeat** at least three times a day.

A THYME INFUSION WITH HONEY

Honey and other products that the hive produces have a lot to offer people who suffer from nose and throat problems, and are particularly good for sore throats. Honey is at the top of the list for its soothing effect. Add it to thyme, which is known for its antimicrobial and anti-inflammatory properties, for a truly effective natural remedy.

TRY IT!
- **Bring a large cup of water to the boil.** As soon as it begins to boil, remove from the heat and add ½ tablespoon of dried thyme. Leave to infuse for 5 minutes, then filter and drink.
- **Add a spoonful of honey** (preferably thyme, rosemary or pine honey), then sip gently, bathing your throat before swallowing.
- **Drink three cups a day.**

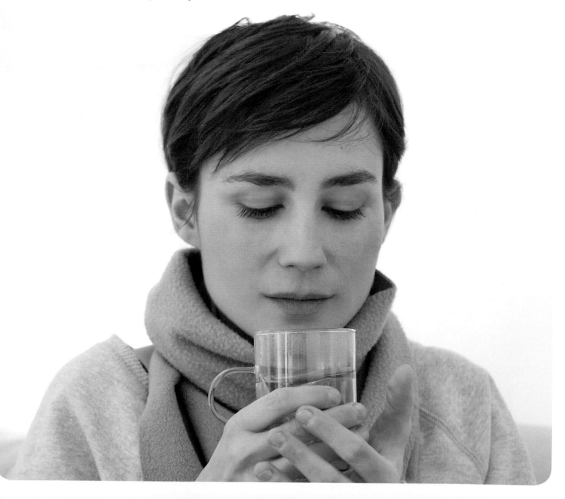

EARACHE

The ear is a complex structure. The external part sends sound through a canal that leads into the eardrum; this transmits the vibration, via the delicate apparatus of the inner ear, to the auditory nerve, which sends the information to the brain. The more complex a system is, the more fragile it is, and such is the case with our ears. Fortunately, earache is usually due to inflammation of the ear canal and eardrum – known as otitis externa, or swimmer's ear. In these instances, natural remedies are usually sufficient to solve the problem. Sometimes an infection develops behind the eardrum, however, which requires more specific care from a medical specialist. This is known as otitis media (middle ear infection). The infections of the inner ear (otitis interna) are more serious, but much rarer.

A GOOD HOT-WATER BOTTLE

Simply applying heat can provide rapid relief to earache. The result may not be long-lasting and the treatment doesn't deal with the cause of the pain, but it would be a shame to deprive yourself of relief that's so easy to obtain!

TRY IT!
- **Get hold of a rubber hot-water bottle**, if possible with a fabric cover, or (if not) wrapped in a towel.
- **Fill it with very hot water,** then place it on your pillow and lie down on the side of the aching ear, with your head on the heat source.
- **Repeat** as often as necessary.

THREE HOMEOPATHIC REMEDIES

This treatment helps to control otitis in its early stages. Begin it as soon as you feel pain in your ear rather than waiting for the pain to become intense. If you don't see any result after 48 hours, see a doctor.

TRY IT!
- **Buy** some granules of Belladonna 9C, Capsicum 9C and Ferrum phosphoricum 9C from a homeopathic remedy supplier.
- **Take 3 granules** every hour, alternating the three products, until the pain stops.

A MASSAGE OIL

Essential oils are effective in both treating the infection and calming the inflammation that cause the pain. These mixtures will provide you with speedy relief. The active ingredients of the plants, concentrated in the essence extracted from them, will penetrate the skin to treat the affected tissues. The pain will generally cease within two to three days. If it continues, see a doctor.

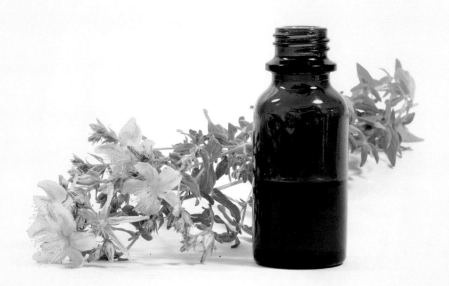

TRY IT!
- Pour 100 ml (3½ fl oz) of St John's wort oil into an opaque or dark-coloured bottle.
- Add 10 drops of eucalyptus essential oil, 10 drops of niaouli essential oil and 10 drops of tea tree essential oil. Stir together well.
- Dab a few drops of the mixture around the affected ear (or ears) and massage in.
- Repeat three times a day until you feel an improvement, then continue for 48 hours after symptoms have disappeared.

SINUS PAIN

The sinuses are cavities, lined with mucous membranes, located in the bone structure of the face: on the forehead, on either side of the nose and above the jaw. The sinuses are connected to the nasal cavities, which have a narrow drainage channel. When this channel becomes inflamed, mucous secretions can block it, leaving germs free to breed in the cosy and welcoming little 'chamber'. This is sinusitis, and the pain it causes can be intense.

AN INHALANT WITH ESSENTIAL OILS

The antiseptic, anti-inflammatory and pain-relieving active ingredients contained in essential oils can be 'carried' by steam into your sinuses. When you inhale the steam, the active ingredients come into direct contact with infected or inflamed mucous membranes. Relief is rapid.

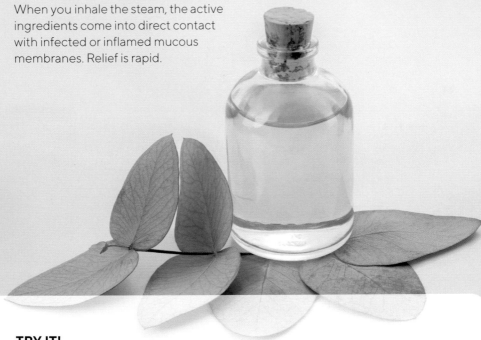

TRY IT!
- **Add 3 drops of eucalyptus essential oil** and 3 drops of peppermint essential oil to a bowl of boiling water.
- **Inhale the steam** emerging from the bowl, breathing in deeply so that your sinuses are bathed in the active ingredients.
- **For maximum effect**, lean over the bowl and cover your head with a towel to form a little 'chamber'.
- **Repeat** three times a day.

MASSAGING THE FOREHEAD, HANDS AND FEET

On your forehead are several energy points related to inflammation of the sinuses. Reflex zones corresponding to these cavities are also located on your hands and feet. You'll need a complete massage!

TRY IT!
- **Start by rubbing your hands** together to warm them up, then massage the tips of the fingers, one by one, starting with the thumb. Do this on both hands.
- **Next, massage the tips of your toes** in the same way.
- **Finally, using your index finger**, stimulate the points on your forehead – first in the centre, between your eyebrows, then at the inner end of your eyebrows (on both sides of your nose) and finally at the centre point of each eyebrow.
- **To improve the effectiveness of this massage**, put a drop of ravintsara essential oil on the tips of your index fingers before massaging these points.
- **Repeat** several times a day.

A MASSAGE WITH ESSENTIAL OILS

All essential oils contain antibacterial substances that penetrate the skin to reach the place where they can be most useful. In addition, some oils are anti-inflammatory and pain relieving. These oils help to control local infection and calm inflammation of the mucous membranes.

TRY IT!
- **Add 2 drops of tea tree essential oil**, 2 drops of niaouli essential oil and 2 drops of thyme essential oil to 1 teaspoonful of calendula oil.
- **Use this mixture** to gently massage the place where the pain is located – on either side of the nose, on the forehead or wherever.
- **Repeat** three times a day until the pain subsides.

④ MUSCLE PAIN

The body contains more than 600 muscles, large and small, of many kinds. Some work independently of our conscious will, like those that allow the digestive tract to contract to push through chewed food. Others are activated by orders we give them. This happens every time you make a movement: you decide to move your arm or to move your hand to grasp an object; the brain passes on the information to the relevant muscles, which contract with the energy needed (neither too much nor too little) to carry out the action. These precious 'striated' muscles sometimes suffer pain, which can be alleviated with simple natural remedies.

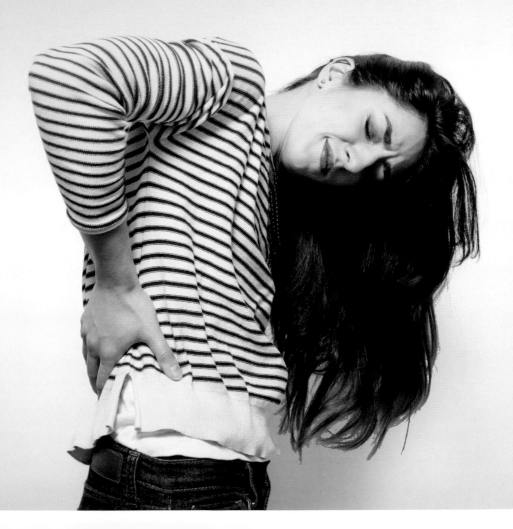

MUSCLE SORENESS

Muscular aches and pains arise after unaccustomed physical effort – for example, when you take up sports again after a holiday, or after you undertake unusually strenuous activity. Such aches usually make themselves known after a few hours of rest, often when you wake up the next day. For a long time, muscle soreness was attributed to an accumulation of lactic acid in the muscle, but this theory has now been rejected. Today, experts speak of muscle microtrauma, which causes microscopic lesions and sometimes ruptures of the tiny blood vessels that pass through the muscles. To quickly alleviate these unpleasant aches and pains, which can last for several days, you'll need to gently work the affected muscle for a few days. A few supplementary treatments will speed up recovery.

A HOT BATH WITH ROSEMARY

Some studies have shown that rosemary may have an anti-inflammatory and pain-relieving effect. Add to a hot bath to alleviate muscle soreness, with the heat promoting the penetration of the plant's active ingredients through the pores of the skin. It also contributes directly to muscle improvement!

TRY IT!
- **Prepare a concentrated infusion of rosemary** by heating 2 litres (3½ pints) of water in a pan. As soon as it boils, remove it from the heat and add 50 g (1¾ oz) of dried rosemary. Leave to infuse for 20 minutes, then filter.
- **Run a fairly hot bath** – about 38°C (100°F) – and pour the rosemary infusion under the running water.
- **Immerse yourself in this fragrant bath** and stay there for at least 15 minutes. Add a little more hot water occasionally, so that the water temperature remains stable.
- **When you get out of the bath**, wrap yourself in a large bathrobe and lie down to give the rosemary time to act.
- **Repeat** daily until the pain subsides.

TWO HOMEOPATHIC REMEDIES

Homeopaths recommend two remedies (see below) for muscle soreness.
Their effectiveness in reducing the pain and inflammation caused by strenuous
physical exercise has been noted by homeopaths for more than two centuries.

TRY IT!

- **Buy** some granules of Rhus toxicodendron 9C and Arnica 5C online from
  a supplier of homeopathic remedies.
- **Take 3 granules of each** (at the same time) three times a day between meals.
- **Repeat** until the pain has completely disappeared.

HOT CLAY POULTICES

Here again, heat is used to accelerate the
disappearance of muscle soreness. But clay
also plays a vital dual role: it 'attracts' waste
that clogs the muscle tissue and contributes
to the soreness, and through the skin it
diffuses minerals that will strengthen
the muscles.

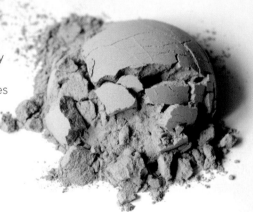

TRY IT!

- **Pour 6 tablespoons of powdered green clay** (8–10 if muscle soreness is
  widespread) into a large bowl.
- **Heat a little water** in a saucepan. As soon as it begins to simmer, pour it very
  gradually into the clay, stirring with a wooden spoon.
- **Stop stirring as soon as a paste forms** – it should be neither too sticky nor
  too firm, and should spread easily without running.
- **Spread this paste** on the sore muscle (be careful not to burn yourself – wait
  1–2 minutes if the paste is too hot) and leave it to work for about 20 minutes.
- **Rinse** in warm water.
- **Repeat** twice a day.

CRAMPS

These sudden, involuntary and painful muscular contractions harden the muscle to the point where it feels like wood. They can occur at rest or when you're moving, and their causes are various – for example, excessive sweating, mineral deficiency or overexertion. The first thing to do when cramp strikes is stretch the muscle in the opposite direction – for example, by flexing your foot if the cramp is in your calf muscle). The cramp will usually ease in less than a minute. If it doesn't, there are some natural remedies that can help to relieve it.

MARINE MAGNESIUM

A deficiency in magnesium is common in Western societies. Almost all of us suffer a nutritional deficiency of this essential mineral, which contributes to more than 200 enzyme-related responses in the body and is involved in the flow of information in the nervous system and the brain. Magnesium deficiency can result in cramps, so if you frequently suffer from them, even when you haven't been involved in unusually strenuous physical activity, you should consider taking magnesium supplements.

TRY IT!

- **Magnesium** is available in many forms – as powder or as tablets, for instance.
- **Choose marine magnesium**, because it's the easiest for the body to assimilate.
- **Follow the packet instructions**, as dosages vary depending on the product. Take it for at least three weeks and repeat every three months. Take care to avoid high doses (more than 400 mg), as this can cause diarrhoea.
- **In addition**, increase your intake of magnesium-rich foods, such as algae, almonds, walnuts, wholegrain rice, spinach, fish and seafood.

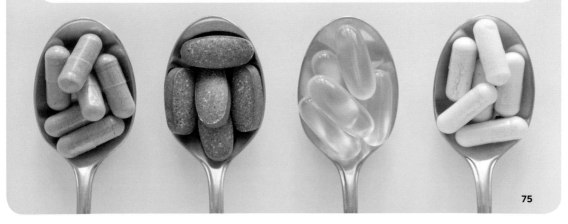

THREE POINTS TO MASSAGE

By stimulating certain energy points, you'll help your muscles to relax and you'll avoid painful cramps. This is a simple remedy that's easy to put into practice in any situation – and it's very fast acting. Use lavender essential oil in the massage for an even speedier recovery.

TRY IT!
- **The first point is on the hand**, in the fleshy part between your thumb and your index finger. To find it, spread out your index finger and thumb and feel for the point located at the bottom of this 'fork', just below the joint.
- **The second point** is on the foot, about two finger-widths below where the first two toes meet.
- **The third point** is located on the shin, where the tibia and fibula meet – about four finger-widths below the kneecap.
- **Pour a drop of lavender essential oil on the tip of your finger and massage these points in order.**
- **Massage each point for 1–2 minutes.** If the cramp persists, start again.

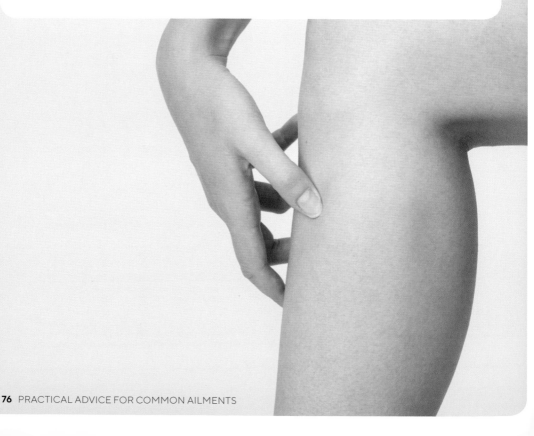

TWO HOMEOPATHIC REMEDIES

Homeopathy provides two drugs (see below) that are very useful if you suffer from occasional cramps – and indispensable when cramps occur frequently. In the first instance, treatment can be a one-off. But in the second, it's best to take the drugs as a course of treatment to prevent recurrence.

TRY IT!

- **Buy** some granules of Cuprum 7C and Nux vomica 7C online from a supplier of homeopathic remedies. Take the granules with you when you're playing sports or working out.
- **When you feel a painful cramp coming on**, take 3 granules of each, at the same time. Repeat an hour later if the cramp persists.
- **If the cramps are recurrent**, continue the treatment, repeating the above dose three times a day for a month.

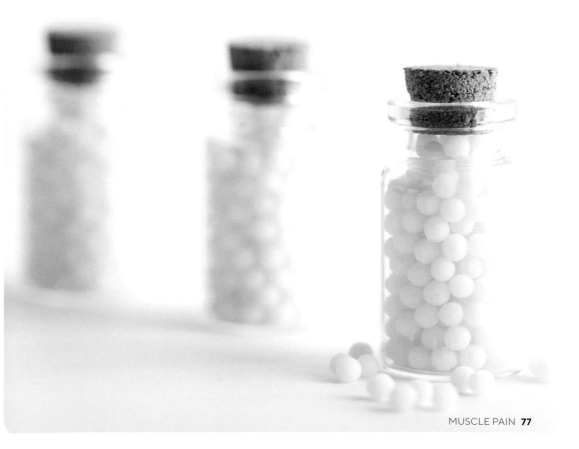

⑤ JOINT PAIN

It's thanks to our joints, of which the body has more than 300, that we can move. Involving all the elements necessary for movement – bones, muscles, tendons and ligaments – they are complex, sensitive and highly efficient systems. It's no wonder, then, that they can be fragile. Sometimes all it takes is a clumsy movement or sleeping in an uncomfortable position for pain to set in, not to mention joint diseases related to cartilage wear and tear, such as osteoarthritis, which we'll discuss further (see page 86).

TENDINITIS

An inflammation of the tendons that attach the muscles to the bones, tendinitis is often linked to a sudden movement that 'pulled' on the tendons, causing microtrauma. It can also be caused by repetitive movements – so golf players may be vulnerable to tendinitis in the shoulder, for example, while tennis players may suffer from pain in the elbow and cyclists from knee problems. Tendinitis is benign, but can sometimes be very disabling. As a first recourse, you should rest the joint (if you're in pain, you may not really have a choice). But you shouldn't remain immobile for too long – you'll need to start moving again, gradually and gently, for the joint tissues to return to full mobility. Certain natural remedies can be a big help.

HOMEOPATHIC GRANULES

This remedy is produced from a very poisonous plant: poison ivy. Fortunately, the extreme dilution of homeopathy neutralizes its toxicity, and what remains is a drug that alleviates pain, reduces fluid retention and calms inflammation.

TRY IT!
- **Buy** some granules of Rhus toxicodendron 9C from a supplier of homeopathic remedies.
- **Take 3 granules**, three times a day, until you're better.

A MASSAGE WITH WINTERGREEN ESSENTIAL OIL

The anti-inflammatory effect of wintergreen is exceptional. Its active ingredients penetrate the skin to heal damaged joint tissues, reducing inflammation and easing pain. It's a simple and practical remedy.

TRY IT!
- **Get hold of** a bottle of wintergreen essential oil.
- **Pour 3–6 drops** (depending on the surface to be covered) onto the painful joint. Massage gently so that the oil penetrates without causing pain.
- **Repeat** as often as necessary (up to six or seven times a day), until the pain subsides.

A COLD CLAY POULTICE WITH WILLOW

Cold reduces the pain of tendinitis. Clay adds its soothing, relaxing, remineralizing and alkalizing properties. Add a pain-relieving plant, willow, and you've got a complete and effective remedy.

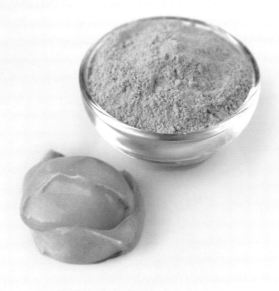

TRY IT!

- **Start by preparing a concentrated willow decoction:** pour 1 tablespoon of dried willow bark into a cup of cold water. Transfer to a pan and bring to the boil, then reduce the heat to a simmer for 15 minutes. Filter the mixture and leave to cool to room temperature, then refrigerate.
- **Pour 6–10 tablespoons of powdered green clay** (depending on the size of the area to be covered) into a large bowl. Gradually add the ice-cold decoction in a thin stream, stirring constantly using a wooden spoon.
- **Stop as soon as you get a paste** that's neither too liquid nor too sticky.
- **Spread this paste** on the painful joint and cover with a piece of gauze. Leave it to work for at least 10 minutes. Rinse in warm water.
- **Repeat** twice a day.

STIFF NECK

Sleeping in a bad position, pulling a muscle or making a sudden movement to look behind you can all cause persistent neck pain. The muscles that cover the delicate cervical structure contract and become painful, sometimes making it impossible to turn your head. The pain can spread to your shoulder and even your back. It may be nothing serious, but it causes discomfort and pain. To dispel the pain, you need to relax the tense muscles and put your trust in natural painkillers.

MASSAGING THE HANDS AND FEET

Reflex zones corresponding to the neck are found on the hands and feet. By massaging them regularly, you'll send an energy message to your neck that will help to relax it.

TRY IT!
- **The reflex zones corresponding to the neck** are on the hand at the base of the thumb and on the foot at the base of the big toe.
- **Massage these areas** several times a day to relax the muscles of your neck.

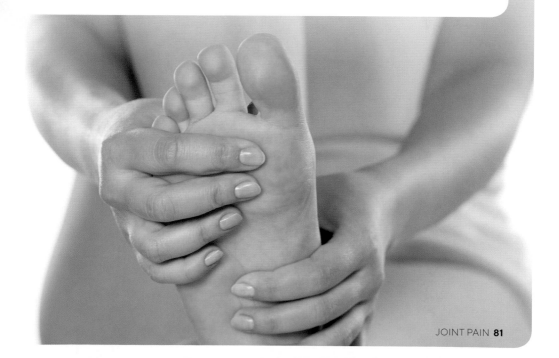

A MASSAGE WITH ROSEMARY AND LAVENDER

The essential oils extracted from these two plants have a relaxing and painkilling effect. They're perfect for dispersing muscular 'knots' and are simple to use.

TRY IT!
- **In an opaque or dark-coloured bottle**, mix equal parts of rosemary camphor essential oil and lavender essential oil.
- **Put 2 or 3 drops of this mixture** onto the painful area.
- **Massage gently** so that the oil penetrates without causing pain.
- **Repeat** three or four times a day until you feel an improvement.

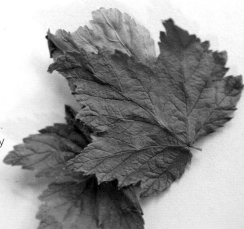

A HOT COMPRESS WITH BLACKCURRANT

Heat is the best remedy for relaxing muscles. Add the pain-relieving and anti-inflammatory action of blackcurrant leaves and you've got the perfect relief for a stiff neck.

TRY IT!
- **Prepare a concentrated infusion of blackcurrant leaves** by pouring 3 tablespoons of the dried leaves into a large bowl of boiling water. Leave it to steep for 15 minutes.
- **Warm this infusion** over a very low heat (don't allow it to boil).
- **Dip a thick cotton cloth** (a piece of towel, for example) into it.
- **Apply the compress to the painful area** and leave it to work until the cloth becomes cool.
- **Repeat** as often as necessary.

BACK PAIN

You use your back, with its fine structure of bones, tendons, ligaments and muscles, in innumerable daily movements. Whether you're bending over, carrying a heavy object or twisting from the waist, you're engaging your back. It's no wonder, then, that it sometimes suffers problems. Also, stress can cause contractures, or permanent shortenings, in all the muscles of the back. A few natural remedies can help to stem these problems before they become serious.

A STEAM BATH AT HOME

Steam baths relieve tension of all kinds, whether nervous or physical. Make the most of them, because back pains are aggravated by stress. If you have a local spa, make regular visits to its steam room. If not, treat yourself to this home remedy, which is made even more effective with the addition of essential oils.

TRY IT!
- **Put a stool or chair** in your bathroom.
- **Pour 10 drops each of rosemary camphor essential oil and pine essential oil** into an essential oil diffuser. Place the diffuser in the bathroom, close the door and let the essences diffuse for about 10 minutes.
- **Set to the highest temperature, turn on the bath taps or shower** and let the water run for a few minutes. Leave the bathroom and close the door to let the steam invade the room.
- **Then simply return to the room, close the door** and sit for at least 5 minutes to soak up the steam and essences. Breathe in deeply so that the active ingredients enter your body, and let the hot steam dissolve the tension in your back.
- **Repeat** as often as necessary.

A HOT BATH WITH HEATHER

Hot baths are a good solution for relieving back pain, because they treat an extended area, reaching places where it's difficult for you to apply treatments. The heat helps to relax tense and contracted muscles, while heather is a traditional aid to relieving muscle and joint pain.

TRY IT!
- **Heat 2 litres (3½ pints) of water** in a saucepan. As soon as it boils, remove from the heat and add a cup of dried heather flowers. Leave to steep for 15 minutes.
- **Meanwhile**, run a hot bath – about 38°C (100°F). When the heather has infused sufficiently, filter out the leaves and add the heather infusion to the bath water.
- **Immerse yourself in the bath** and stay there for at least 20 minutes, adding a little hot water occasionally to prevent it going cold.
- **When you get out of the bath**, wrap yourself in a bathrobe and lie down for 15 minutes, to allow the plant's active ingredients to finish penetrating your skin.
- **You can take a heather bath** regularly if you suffer from chronic pain.

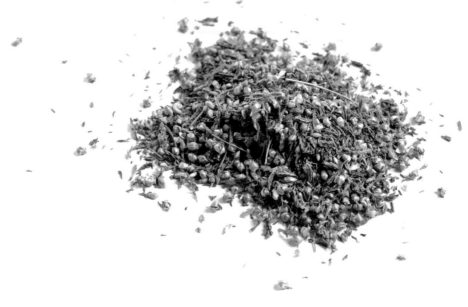

A YOGA POSTURE

Yoga is recommended for reducing pain caused by posture. This stretch improves blood circulation throughout the body and calms the nervous system. It also helps to relieve back pain, while improving overall flexibility.

TRY IT!
- **Stand up**, with your arms by your sides, and your feet parallel and about 1 m (3 ft) apart. Keep your chest straight and facing forwards throughout this exercise.
- **Turn your right foot** in and your left foot out, then stretch over to your left side (without causing yourself any pain).
- **Place your left hand** on your foot (or on your knee if you can't stretch further down). Keeping your right arm straight, lift it to point directly upwards.
- **Lift your head**, looking up towards your right hand.
- **Hold this position** as you count to ten, then go back to your original position and do the exercise on the other side.
- **Repeat** the exercise five times on each side.

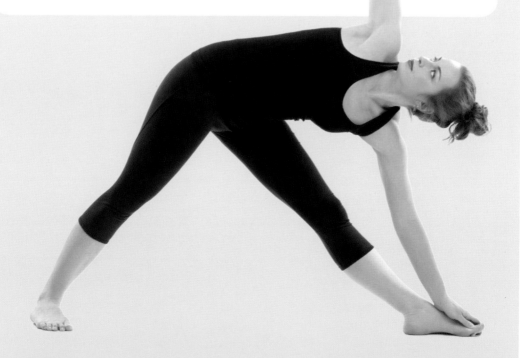

⑥ RHEUMATIC PAINS

Rheumatism, as a term, covers many different conditions. Here we concentrate on the pain associated with osteoarthritis and rheumatoid arthritis. Osteoarthritis is a degenerative disease caused by wear and tear on the joints (the protective cartilage becomes damaged, thus allowing bones to collide painfully), while rheumatoid arthritis is an inflammation of the tissues. Both generally include joint pain, swelling and stiffness. So how can you tell which is which? If your painful joint is white and cold, you probably have osteoarthritis. If it's red and hot, it's more likely rheumatoid arthritis, or osteoarthritis complicated by inflammation. Most natural remedies will help in either case. All anti-inflammatory remedies can help to soothe these conditions when tissues are inflamed (which is very common). Pain-relieving remedies are suitable for all types of rheumatism, with one difference: if your joint is inflamed, choose a cold treatment; if it isn't, it's heat that will soothe you. Compresses, poultices and wraps can therefore be prepared hot or cold, depending on your condition.

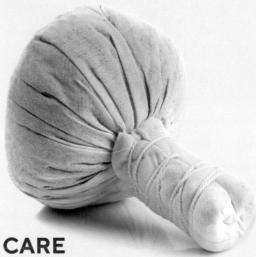

GENERAL CARE

Certain treatments are taken orally and act 'from the inside'. Others, especially baths, can have overall effectiveness despite acting 'from the outside'. All are suitable for all types of painful joints.

A MEADOWSWEET INFUSION

This infusion is particularly effective for relieving pain and calming local inflammation. Meadowsweet appears to inhibit the production of the prostaglandins that cause inflammation. As a bonus, the plant is slightly diuretic, which promotes the elimination of waste from the kidneys.

TRY IT!

- **The flowering tops of meadowsweet plants are used in infusions**, with or without the leaves. Drink two or three cups a day.
- **Add ½ tablespoon of the dried plant** to a large cup of just-boiled water. Leave it to steep for 5 minutes.
- **You can also** consume meadowsweet in the form of plant powder (in capsules).

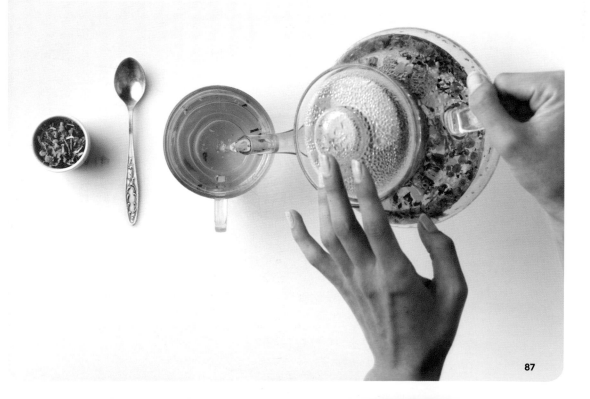

DEVIL'S CLAW EXTRACT

If there's one essential plant for people suffering from
rheumatism, this is surely it! Devil's claw stimulates the
renewal of cartilage and strengthens it; and the plant also has
a pain-relieving effect, due mainly to its anti-inflammatory action.

TRY IT!

- **The simplest way to take devil's claw** is in easy-to-use products such as plant
  powder (in capsules), liquid extracts (in a dropper bottle) and mother tincture
  (also in a dropper bottle). This last form is the most suitable if you suffer from
  digestive problems.
- **Devil's claw** can also be brewed in a decoction. Add ½ tablespoon of dried
  root to a bowl of cold water. Leave to soak for 4 hours, then bring to the boil.
  Remove from the heat and leave to infuse for 10 minutes.
- **Drink** two cups a day, between meals.

A WINTERGREEN AND PEPPERMINT MASSAGE

Whether carried out on a joint that covers a large area, such as a shoulder or
knee, or a much smaller one, such as a wrist or finger, this massage will produce
good results. Wintergreen is a powerful anti-inflammatory, while peppermint
is a fast-working pain reliever.

TRY IT!

- **Mix 2 parts of wintergreen essential oil with 1 part of peppermint essential oil**
  in an opaque or dark-coloured bottle.
- **Pour 2–5 drops** (depending on the surface area to be covered) onto the
  painful joint.
- **Massage** to penetrate the essential oil into the joint.
- **Repeat** three times a day until the swelling subsides and the pain disappears.

THREE MASSAGE POINTS ON YOUR WRIST

Whichever wrist joint is affected, massaging these three points, situated on the energy meridians of traditional Chinese medicine, will help to relieve your pain. By rebalancing the energy circulating in your body, you can reduce the number of painful inflammatory episodes you suffer.

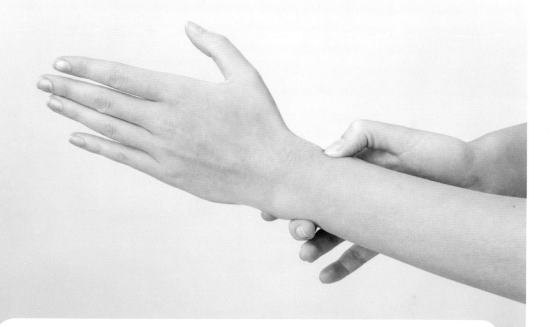

TRY IT!
- **To find the first point**, follow the edge of your thumb right down to the base of the joint, where the wrist bends. The point is located two finger-widths below that.
- **The second point** is also on your wrist, but this time on the inside. Find the crease at the base of your palm. From the mid-point, measure two finger-widths down and the point is there, between the bones you can feel under the skin.
- **The third point** is located a little lower, one extra finger-width below (that is, three finger-widths below the wrist crease).
- **Massage these points** with the thumb of the opposite hand, first in one direction, then in the other (1 minute in each direction).
- **Do the same massage** on both wrists, and repeat four or five times a day.

TREATMENTS FOR SMALL JOINTS

Certain remedies are very effective on small joints but are difficult to perform on larger ones. Make the most of these if the pain is in your wrist, fingers or ankles, for example.

A CHILLI POULTICE

Capsaicin, which gives chillies their hot flavour, can be taken orally, in food (see page 25), but also administered locally to alleviate pain. You can find various capsaicin products on the market, including plasters and ointments, but you can also prepare your own poultice at home.

TRY IT!
- **Choose chillies** that are not too pungent, so that your skin will tolerate the heat they produce.
- **Very finely mince or blend enough fresh chillies (green or red) to make 1–2 tablespoons of paste.** Mix this with a few drops of warm water to make it more fluid, but without it becoming liquid.
- **Spread the mixture over a square of gauze**, then cover with another square of gauze to form a small poultice.
- **Apply this on the painful joint** and hold it in place with an elastic bandage. Leave it to work for about 20 minutes, then rinse with warm water.
- **If the poultice** causes a disagreeable burning sensation, remove it, as it means the chilli is too strong for your skin. Go through the process again with a less fiery type of chilli or dilute the minced chilli paste.

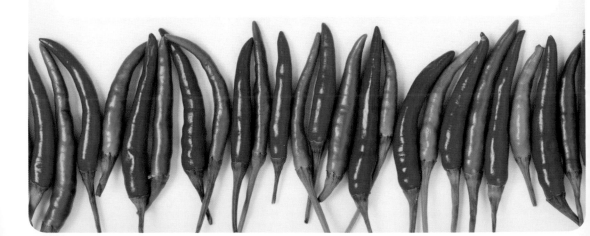

AN ONION-JUICE COMPRESS

Onion contains anti-inflammatory and painkilling substances that act locally.
One onion is enough to make an easy compress to relieve small joints.

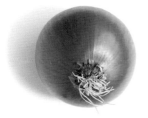 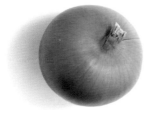 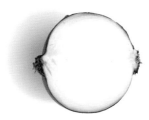

TRY IT!
- **Put one white onion** (or half, if the joint you want to treat is very small) in a blender and mix into a puree.
- **Filter the onion puree** through a fine strainer or a piece of fine muslin, and reserve the juice.
- **Soak a cotton cloth** in this juice, then place it on the painful joint. Hold it in place with an elastic bandage.
- **Leave it to work** for at least 1 hour, then rinse with warm or lukewarm water.

A VINEGAR COMPRESS

Vinegar has many healing qualities: it neutralizes the acidity of tissues, soothes pain and drains toxins. In addition to being taken orally, it can be used in local applications. You can use hot or cold vinegar, depending on the condition of your joints.

TRY IT!
- **Mix 150 ml (5¼ fl oz) water and 150 ml (5¼ fl oz) apple cider vinegar.**
- **Chill this mixture** before using it on joints that are red, hot and swollen. Alternatively, if your joints are white and cold, heat the mixture gently first.
- **Soak a cotton cloth in the mixture.**
- **Apply it on the affected joint.** Hold it in place for about 20 minutes.
- **Repeat** until the pain decreases.

TREATMENTS FOR LARGE JOINTS

Some treatments won't be practical for large areas such as shoulders, knees and elbows. On the other hand, other external remedies work very well on them.

A LEMON-EUCALYPTUS CLAY WRAP

Clay wraps are effective on many levels. First, a hot or cold wrap (depending on how you prepare it) soothes the joint tissues. The clay eliminates their waste and recharges them with minerals. The lemon eucalyptus essential oil adds an anti-inflammatory and painkilling action. All joints, even large ones, can benefit from this treatment.

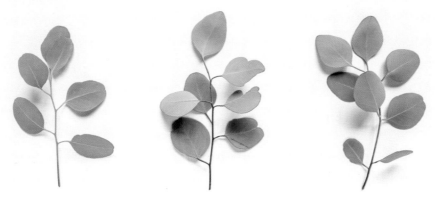

TRY IT!
- Put 5–10 tablespoons of green clay powder (or more, depending on the area to be covered) into a bowl.
- Add 3–6 drops of lemon eucalyptus essential oil.
- Warm up some water in a saucepan or cool it in the refrigerator, depending on whether you want a hot or cold wrap.
- Gradually add the water to the clay in a thin stream, stirring with a wooden spoon.
- Stop when the clay has the consistency of thick cream (neither too sticky nor too liquid).
- Spread the clay in a thick layer over the joint, then wrap in an elastic bandage.
- Leave to work for at least 30 minutes, then rinse with warm water.
- Repeat two or three times a day.

A HOT-WATER BOTTLE OR AN ICE PACK

It's not easy to put a hot-water bottle or ice bag on a finger or toe. But both are much easier to use to relieve pain in an elbow, knee or shoulder. Here, again, choose heat or cold depending on the appearance of your painful joint. If you're in doubt, try it and see: how you feel will tell you quickly what sort of joint problem you have. This very simple remedy is a perfect complement to other treatments.

TRY IT!
- **Fill a hot-water bottle**, or get an ice pack out of the freezer (or fill a plastic bag with ice).
- **Wrap the hot-water bottle or ice pack** in a cotton cloth, then place it on the painful joint.
- **Leave in place** until the hot-water bottle or ice pack has returned to room temperature.
- **Repeat** as often as necessary.

MASSAGING THE HANDS AND FEET

To naturally relieve rheumatic pains (especially if they involve large areas that make local treatments more difficult), you can massage reflex zones to stimulate the activity of glands that naturally secrete cortisol, which is both anti-inflammatory and analgesic. These zones are found on the palms of the hands and the soles of the feet.

TRY IT!
- **Start with your feet.** Pour 2 or 3 drops of black spruce essential oil into the palm of your hands, then lightly rub them to distribute the essence.
- **Massage the whole of your soles** (one foot after the other), then focus on two areas: the one in the centre of the arch (which corresponds to the adrenal glands, just above your kidneys) and the one below your big toe (the reflex zone for the parathyroid glands in your neck).
- **Next, do the same with your hands**, focusing on the top of the fleshy mound on the palm below the thumb, and on the base of the thumb.
- **Repeat** as often as necessary.

⑦ INJURY-RELATED PAIN

Life is no bed of roses! Everyday activities sometimes result in accidents that, although generally minor, can have painful consequences. Bangs, burns and falls – they all hurt! Fortunately, natural remedies are there to accelerate healing and eliminate pain.

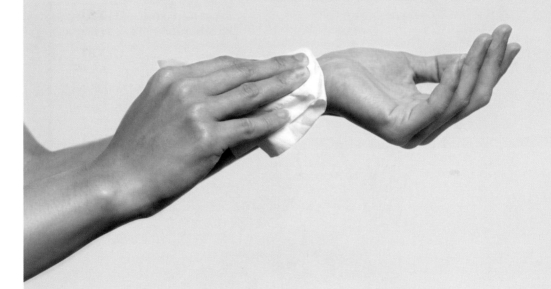

BUMPS AND BRUISES

When you receive a bump, the skin sometimes resists and doesn't break. Over the next few days, the area that has suffered the trauma turns red, then blue, purple and finally a greenish yellow, before returning to normal. It's what's called a haematoma (a bruise), and it's painful to the touch. When the region doesn't change colour but still swells, doctors call it a contusion. The distinction, though, isn't always so straightforward, because contusions often turn blue. Most bumps and bruises are benign and will disappear after eight to ten days without treatment. But some treatments can speed up the progress.

HOMEOPATHIC GRANULES

Arnica comes to the rescue! It's the plant for bumps and the ultimate weapon against bruises.

TRY IT!
- **Always keep** a supply of Arnica 5C at home.
- **In cases of bumps or bruises**, take 5 granules immediately.
- **Repeat** 2 hours later (up to three or four times in all).
- **If you received a bad shock** when you were injured (as a result of a fall, for example), alternate the 5 granules of Arnica 5C with the same of Arnica 15C. The first has a physical effect, while the second also calms the emotions.

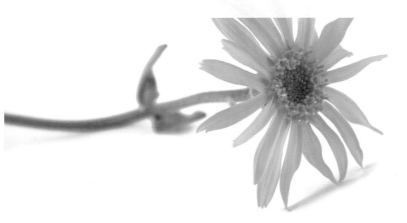

AN ICED LEMON JUICE COMPRESS

If there's nothing else to hand, take a look around your kitchen to see if you have a lemon. This will provide you with a quick and effective remedy, as the lemon will rapidly improve blood circulation in the injured area.

TRY IT!
- **Squeeze a lemon** and immediately wet a cotton pad with the juice.
- **Put the pad in the freezer** for about 10 minutes, then place it on the affected area.
- **Hold it in place for about 20 minutes.** Repeat as often as necessary.
- **This remedy is highly effective** when applied immediately after a knock, before bruising has set in.

HELICHRYSUM ESSENTIAL OIL

This essential oil rapidly reduces bumps and bruises. The treatment is also very straightforward, so make the most of it.

TRY IT!

- **Put 2 or 3 drops of helichrysum essential oil** on the area that has suffered the shock (this essential oil isn't irritating) and rub it in very gently (don't massage).
- **Repeat** three or four times a day, until all traces of bruising disappear.

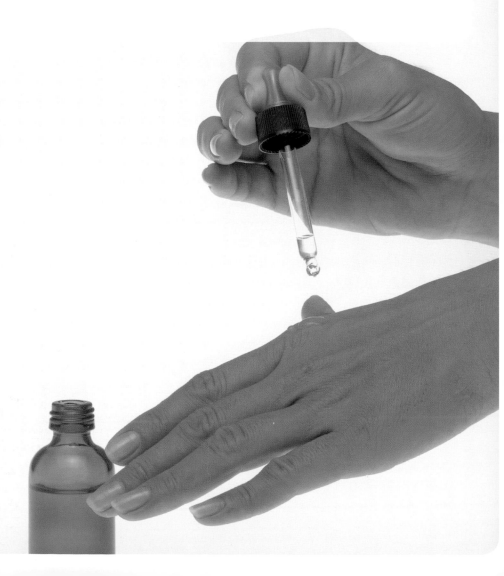

BURNS AND SUNBURN

Many daily activities bring us close to a source of heat. Whether you're ironing or taking a dish out of the oven, it takes only one false move for your skin to come into contact with sufficient heat to damage the tissues. Burns can be very painful. The same is true of serious sunburn, which is a genuine burn and should be treated as such. Burns can be more or less severe, ranging from a simple but painful redness to deep-tissue injuries. Only first-degree burns (when the skin becomes red) or superficial second-degree ones (when the skin forms a painful blister) can be treated at home. If tissue damage is more severe, seek medical attention.

A HONEY POULTICE

Some studies suggest that honey has strong antiseptic and healing properties. It shouldn't, however, be used any which way. Choose an organic honey and keep the jar tightly closed when not in use.

TRY IT!
- **Spread a generous layer** of honey on the burned area and cover with a dressing or a sterile compress covered with an elastic bandage. If the skin is torn, disinfect the area before treating it with honey.
- **Leave to work for 2 hours**, then rinse with warm water.
- **Repeat** three times a day.

LAVENDER ASPIC ESSENTIAL OIL

This essential oil is exceptionally healing, accelerating the regeneration of tissue damaged by burning. As well as pain relieving, it's also antibacterial, which is useful in avoiding secondary infection when the skin is broken.

TRY IT!
- **Pour a few drops of lavender aspic essential oil** on the burn and rub it in very gently.
- **Repeat** every 15 minutes for 1 hour, then repeat three times a day for between five and six days.

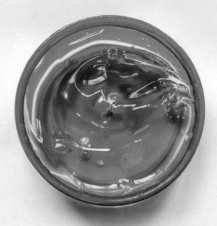

ALOE VERA GEL

Extracted from the fleshy leaves of the large Mediterranean aloe vera plant, this pain-relieving gel has a great affinity with skin, regenerating, healing and nourishing it. In short, the gel has what it takes to quickly relieve burns and accelerate the regeneration of damaged tissue.

TRY IT!

- **Spread a thin layer** of organic aloe vera gel on the burn and leave it to penetrate the skin.
- **Repeat every hour**, then space the applications further as the pain begins to ebb.

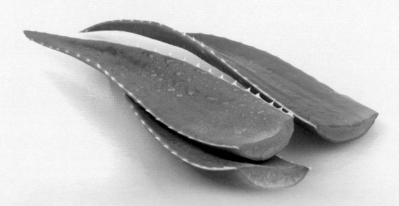

SPRAINS

A sprain is a painful trauma to a joint, caused by an impact, a fall or overstraining of a muscle. It usually affects the joints of the limbs: fingers, ankles, knees, wrists, elbows or, more rarely, shoulders. The ligaments, the strips of connective tissue that hold the bones together, are distorted, stretched or even, in the most severe cases, ruptured. The slightest movement then becomes painful. If a sprain occurs, the joint must first be immobilized – the time varying according to the severity of the sprain. In all cases, some simple remedies can supplement this crucial measure.

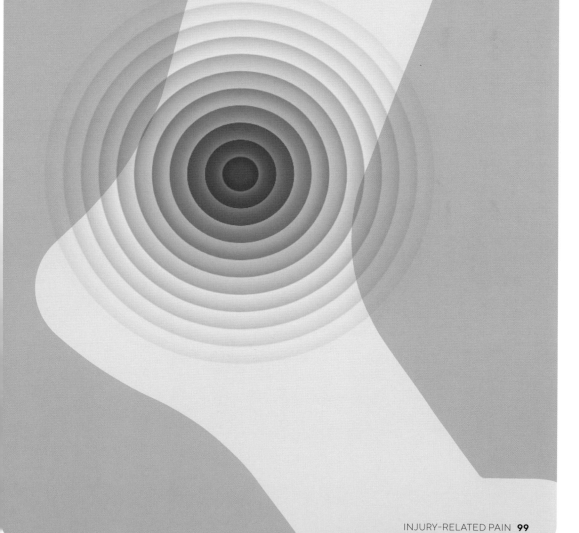

AN ICE PACK

A cure as old as the hills, and still extremely effective, cold helps to neutralize pain and reduce oedema (swelling of tissue). It's the first step to take before all other treatments.

TRY IT!
- **If you have an ice pack**, place it on the affected joint.
- **Alternatively, fill a small plastic bag with ice cubes**, close it and wrap it in a towel before placing it on the joint.
- **Renew the application** as often as necessary.

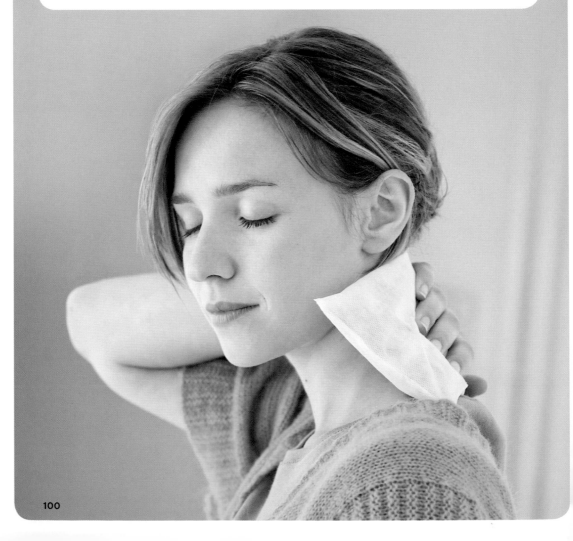

A HOMEOPATHIC REMEDY

As you now know, arnica is a plant renowned for its effectiveness in treating bumps and bruises. It's used in homeopathic medicine as a great remedy for injuries and their physical and psycho-emotional repercussions – and sprains are no exception. The homeopathic dilution of arnica accelerates tissue recovery and provides help in coming to terms with the fear experienced at the time of a fall or accident.

TRY IT!
- **Buy some Arnica 5C and Arnica 15C granules** from a supplier of homeopathic remedies.
- **Take 3 granules** of Arnica 5C every hour during the first 24 hours, then every 3 hours for five days.
- **If the accident has caused intense and lasting fear**, take 3 granules of Arnica 15C at the same time. It works at a deeper and more psycho-emotional level.

A MASSAGE WITH HELICHRYSUM ESSENTIAL OIL

Helichrysum italicum, a flower that's often used in dried-flower arrangements, yields an essential oil that combats bruising, aids circulation and has anti-inflammatory and pain-relieving properties. As well as treating bruises and bumps, the oil also relieves the symptoms of sprains, so take advantage of it!

TRY IT!
- **Put 2–5 drops of helichrysum essential oil** (depending on the size of the joint) on the painful area.
- **Rub in very lightly** so that the oil penetrates without causing pain.
- **Repeat** three times a day until the pain and swelling subside.

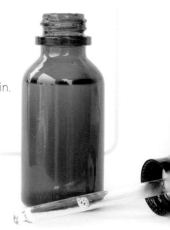

⑧ CARDIOVASCULAR PAIN

Blood circulates continuously in our bodies, propelled through a network of arteries, veins and capillaries to 'deliver' oxygen and essential nutrients to our cells. Next, the blood takes care of metabolic waste and returns to the lungs, then to the heart. This cardiovascular system of heart and blood vessels is a continuous circuit that, like all our biological systems, sometimes malfunctions. Some related conditions are serious and need to be treated in a medical environment. Other, less serious conditions can still be chronic and painful. These include haemorrhoids and heavy legs, which can both benefit from natural remedies.

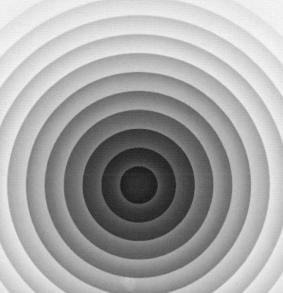

HAEMORRHOIDS

These swollen veins in or around the anus can be very painful. Haemorrhoids (or piles) are sometimes external (when they're visible to the naked eye), sometimes internal (inside the anal canal). In all cases, they cause a feeling of heaviness, itching and painful inflammation. Certain localized remedies can help to alleviate suffering and accelerate healing.

A MASSAGE WITH MASTIC ESSENTIAL OIL

Pistacia lentiscus, the mastic shrub or tree, yields an essential oil that decongests the venous system and stimulates blood circulation that has been disturbed by haemorrhoids. It's also antispasmodic, which helps to alleviate pain.

TRY IT!
- **In the morning**, prepare your massage oil for the day.
- **Mix 10 drops of mastic essential oil** with 1 tablespoon of St John's wort oil (or vegetable oil) and pour into a small opaque or dark-coloured bottle.
- **After using the toilet (passing a stool) or taking a bath or shower**, dip your finger in the oil mixture and gently coat the haemorrhoid.
- **Repeat** for several days, until the problem clears up.

A GINKGO BILOBA CURE

Ginkgo is a plant that's often prescribed to relieve haemorrhoids. It strengthens the tone of the venous walls and regulates blood circulation – a real help if you suffer regularly from haemorrhoids.

TRY IT!
- **Ginkgo** isn't consumed as an infusion, but you'll find the plant extracts (available in capsule or tablet form, or as drops or gel) very effective.
- **During a flare-up**, choose a fairly concentrated product (ask your pharmacist for advice). Follow the packet instructions, as each product is dosed differently. Continue the treatment until the pain stops.
- **If you often suffer from haemorrhoids**, you can take a less concentrated extract as a three-week treatment once every three months.

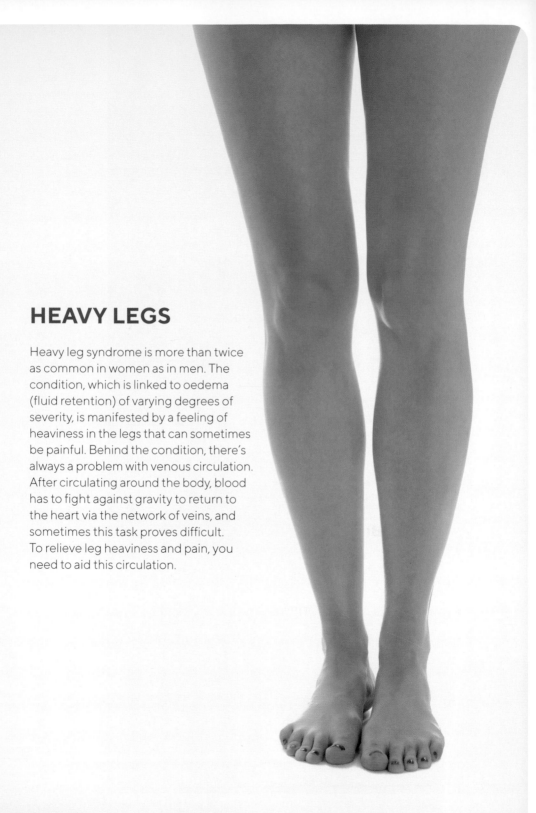

HEAVY LEGS

Heavy leg syndrome is more than twice as common in women as in men. The condition, which is linked to oedema (fluid retention) of varying degrees of severity, is manifested by a feeling of heaviness in the legs that can sometimes be painful. Behind the condition, there's always a problem with venous circulation. After circulating around the body, blood has to fight against gravity to return to the heart via the network of veins, and sometimes this task proves difficult. To relieve leg heaviness and pain, you need to aid this circulation.

A SWEET CLOVER INFUSION

Sweet clover (*Melilotus*) is a traditional natural remedy for combating heavy legs. Research has suggested its effectiveness as an anti-inflammatory and as a treatment for poor circulation and lymphatic blockages. It's a potent weapon against heavy legs!

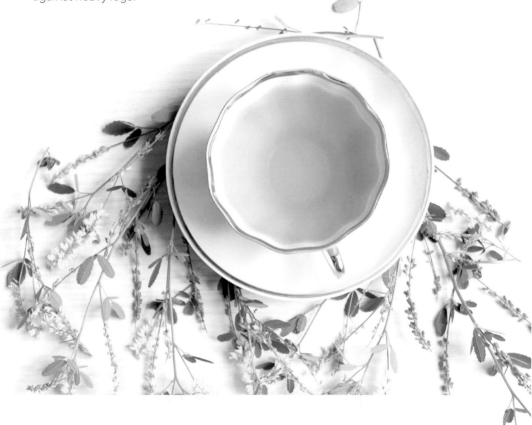

TRY IT!

- **In the morning,** prepare your infusion for the day by adding 1 tablespoonful of dried sweet clover to 1 litre (1¾ pints) of boiling water. Leave to steep for 15 minutes before filtering.
- **Drink this infusion** in small quantities throughout the day. Repeat daily for three weeks. If you need to continue the treatment, leave a two-week gap before starting again.
- **Here, again**, you can use this infusion to soak compresses to put on your legs in the evening.

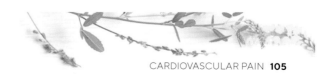

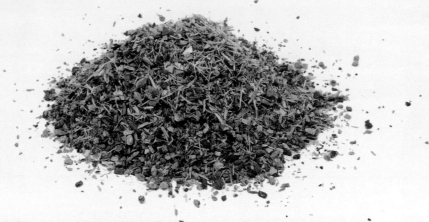

HORSE CHESTNUT BARK

Horse chestnut has been used for centuries to improve venous circulation. Liquid extract of horse chestnut, available in dropper bottles, is effective when taken orally. It can be taken as a course of treatment for at least three weeks. If you're able to get hold of dried horse chestnut bark, try preparing the compress below for soothing relief.

TRY IT!
- **Add 2 tablespoons** of dried bark to 500 ml (17½ fl oz) of cold water.
- **Bring to the boil**, then boil for 10 minutes before filtering.
- **Use this decoction to soak compresses** and place these on your legs in the evening.
- **For a long-lasting effect**, repeat the treatment every evening for at least ten days.

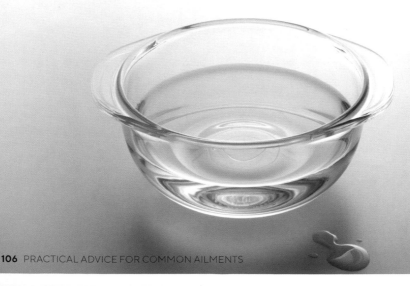

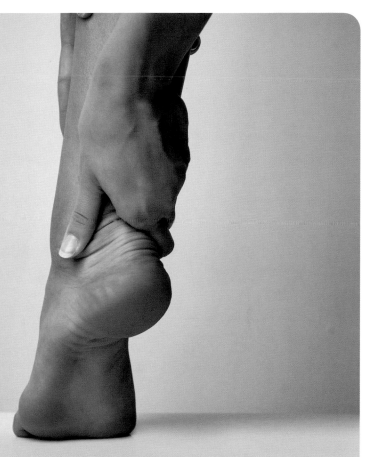

A MASSAGE WITH ESSENTIAL OILS

This treatment includes the essential oils of cypress, which stimulates blood circulation, and juniper, which reinforces the venous walls. It also adds the freshness of peppermint, to provide an immediate feeling of relief.

TRY IT!

- **Pour 100 ml (3½ fl oz) of arnica oil** into an opaque or dark-coloured bottle. Add 20 drops of cypress essential oil, 20 drops of peppermint essential oil and 20 drops of juniper essential oil.
- **Massage your legs with this oil**, morning and evening, always massaging from the bottom to the top of your legs.
- **Focus your attention** on the ankles, if they are swollen, then on the calves, knees and finally thighs.
- **Continue this treatment twice a day** for three weeks. If the symptoms return, repeat the course of treatment after a gap of a month.

9 FEMALE PAINS

A woman's life is marked by cycles dictated by hormonal secretions. And all that involves problems – more for some women than for others. It's unfair, but that's how it is! Menstrual pain, in particular, can be intense for some, while others find that their breasts swell and become painful during their cycle. Certain natural remedies can be a big help.

PERIOD PAIN

Some women experience severe pain in the lower abdomen during the first few days of their periods. This pain can spread to the lower back and evolve into spasms. For those who suffer from painful menstruation, the pain is accompanied by a feeling of discomfort, nausea and headaches. Natural solutions do exist.

A GOOD HOT-WATER BOTTLE

Despite its simplicity, this old remedy gives excellent results. Heat relieves cramps and spasms, so take advantage of it.

TRY IT!
- **Fill a hot-water bottle** with very hot water. If the bottle doesn't have a cover, wrap it in a towel.
- **Lie down in a quiet place** and place the hot-water bottle on your belly. Leave it there until it starts to go cold.
- **Repeat** as often as necessary.
- **Heat also increases the effectiveness** of other painkilling treatments.

A MASSAGE WITH TARRAGON

A herb commonly used in cooking, tarragon is also a true medicinal herb with many healing properties. The essential oil extracted from it is highly antispasmodic, but also anti-inflammatory and pain relieving – a winning combination!

TRY IT!
- **Put 3 drops of pure tarragon essential oil on your lower abdomen** (it's not irritating).
- **Massage to penetrate**, and leave the oil to work, ideally while you relax in a quiet place.
- **Repeat every hour** until the pain subsides.

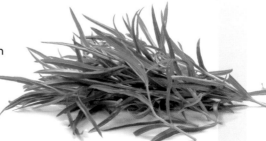

A FEVERFEW INFUSION

Aspirin isn't recommended for relieving menstrual pain, because it increases bleeding. The same applies to pain-relieving plants that contain salicylic compounds, notably meadowsweet and willow bark. Fortunately, feverfew, with its legendary painkilling properties, makes a good substitute.

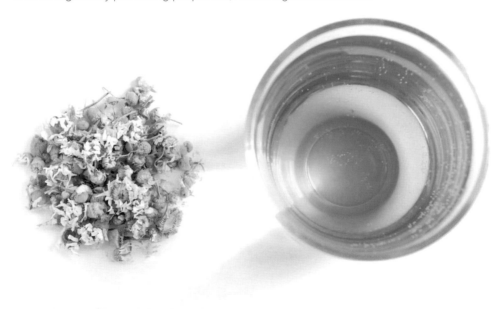

TRY IT!
- **Prepare an infusion** by adding ½ tablespoon of the dried plant to a large cup of boiling water. Leave to steep for 5 minutes before filtering.
- **Drink** in small sips.
- **Repeat** 2 hours later if the pain persists. Drink up to four large cups a day.

BREAST PAINS

Some women, just before a period, find that their breasts swell and become hard and painful. The process isn't clearly understood, but it appears to be due to hormonal variations typical of this stage of the menstrual cycle. However, it's known that during the second half of the cycle, oestrogen production falls and progesterone levels increase, before falling if the egg has not been fertilized. These fluctuations might explain pains in the breasts. Whatever the cause of the pain, natural remedies exist that can help to ease the discomfort.

CHASTEBERRY CAPSULES

The chasteberry fruit (from the tree *Vitex agnus-castus*) combines several healing properties. It has the same effect on the body as progesterone, so compensates for the sudden drop of this hormone just before menstruation. Overall, it balances hormonal production and also inhibits the production of prolactin, which contributes to breast swelling.

TRY IT!
- **Chasteberries can be consumed in dried, powdered form** (as capsules).
- **Follow the packet instructions**, as each product is dosed differently.
- **Repeat** the treatment every month for about ten days, starting a week before your period is due.

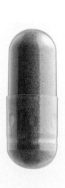
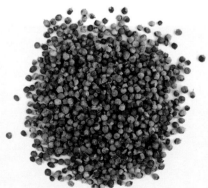

ICE PACKS

Cold compresses are extremely effective in relieving oedema, which causes the breasts to swell, and in soothing the pain. It would be a shame to miss out on this simple remedy!

TRY IT!
- **Wet some cotton cloths** (pieces of towelling, for example).
- **Put them in the freezer** for about 10 minutes.
- **Apply them to the breasts**, leaving them in place until they reach room temperature.
- **Repeat** as often as necessary.

CABBAGE POULTICES

Cabbage contains anti-inflammatory substances that also act locally. It can soothe both oedema and pain.

TRY IT!
- **Spread some large cabbage leaves** on your kitchen worktop, then crush them with a rolling pin to break the veins of the leaves and extract the juice.
- **Place the crushed leaves on your sore breasts** and hold them in place with an elastic bandage.
- **Leave in place for 2 hours.**
- **Repeat** two or three times a day.

DIGESTIVE PROBLEMS

FLATULENCE

This is an accumulation of air in the stomach. You feel bloated, the stomach wall is tight and the upper part of the abdomen is hard to the touch. Air can be swallowed while eating – for example, while chewing gum, slurping soup that's too hot to swallow or drinking too many fizzy drinks. Flatulence can also be the result of eating too quickly, as this means you swallow a lot of air with each mouthful (excessive air swallowing is known as aerophagia). Stress also seems to play a role. Certain natural remedies can help you to get rid of the air that causes pain.

A THREE-SPICE INFUSION
Cumin, caraway and fennel seeds are all carminative – meaning they help to evacuate air trapped in the stomach. They also aid digestion, so are doubly effective in relieving flatulence.

TRY IT!
- **Prepare a mixture** of equal parts of fennel, caraway and cumin seeds.
- **Add 1 tablespoon** of the mixture to a large cup of boiling water and leave to steep for 5 minutes, then filter and drink.
- **Drink a cup** when the symptoms become apparent, and repeat 1 hour later if the trouble persists.
- **If you regularly suffer from flatulence**, drink a cup after your two main meals of the day for at least ten days.

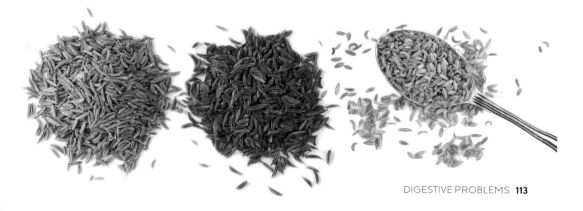

ACTIVATED CHARCOAL

This is pure powdered carbon, made from wood, peat or other carbon sources. It's filled with small cells, which give the substance great absorbing capacity. When you swallow activated charcoal, it attracts and traps both the gases and the toxins in the stomach. As it's neither digested nor metabolized, the charcoal, loaded with what it has absorbed as it passes through the digestive tract, is passed in stools.

TRY IT!
- **You can use activated charcoal occasionally**, whenever you feel discomfort. Take a dose of the powder with a glass of water (follow the packet instructions for the correct dosage).
- **Repeat** 2 hours later if symptoms persist.
- **If you regularly suffer from flatulence**, take one dose mid-morning and another mid-afternoon for a period of ten days.
- **Activated charcoal** is also effective in ridding the body of intestinal gas (see opposite).

GINGER VINEGAR

Apple cider vinegar, which is less acidic than wine vinegar, has an alkalizing effect on the digestive system, helping to reduce excess stomach acidity. Ginger helps to neutralize and expel gas. Together, they make a powerful flatulence antidote.

TRY IT!
- **Peel a 50 g piece of ginger,** cut it into pieces and add to a 250 ml (½ pint) bottle or jar. Fill with organic cider vinegar, seal and leave for ten days in a cool, dark place.
- **If you're prone to flatulence**, add 1 tablespoon of this vinegar to your diet every day – for example, to season salads.
- **At times when flatulence is a particular problem**, dilute 1 tablespoon of the vinegar in a glass of water at room temperature and drink immediately.
- **Repeat 2 hours later** if symptoms persist.
- **You can follow the same procedure** if you know you're going to be eating foods that encourage the production of gas, such as cabbages and legumes.

BLOATING

A difficulty in properly breaking down foods before they enter the intestine can result in an accumulation of gases in the intestine, leading to a bloated feeling. To neutralize or evacuate these unwanted gases, you'll therefore need to work on the whole digestive system. Stress is an aggravating factor. A diet too rich in fibre can also cause bloating in people with fragile intestines. When you're feeling bloated, try these simple remedies.

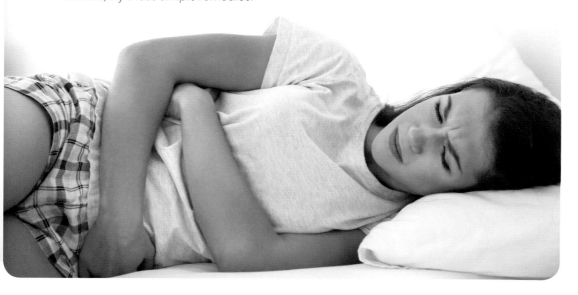

A BELLY MASSAGE

Simple massage strokes can help the intestine to evacuate the excess gas it contains. Essential oils add digestive and pain-relieving properties.

TRY IT!

- **Prepare a massage oil** by adding 2 drops of tarragon essential oil and 2 drops of basil essential oil to 2 tablespoons of vegetable oil. Mix well.
- **Use this oil to massage your belly**, moving your hands around your navel in a clockwise direction.
- **Massage slowly for 10 minutes**, keeping your strokes moderate to avoid intensifying the unpleasant sensation.
- **Repeat** 2 hours later if symptoms persist.

CLAY MILK

Clay is highly absorbent. As it moves through the digestive tract, it 'grabs' the excess air and the toxins that have accumulated there. Then, as clay isn't digested, it exits the body with them.

TRY IT!
- **Pour 1 tablespoon** of white clay powder into a glass of water at room temperature. Leave to rest for 10 minutes.
- **Stir and drink.**
- **If you are prone to constipation**, don't stir the mixture, and drink only the water (not the clay at the bottom of the glass).

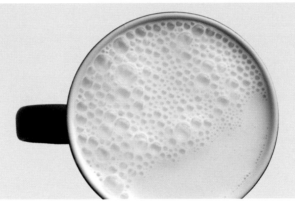

TARRAGON ESSENTIAL OIL

This essential oil promotes digestion and combats the intestinal fermentation of certain foods that produce a lot of gas.

TRY IT!
- **When you're feeling bloated**, add 1 drop of tarragon essential oil to 1 teaspoon of honey, and swallow.
- **If you're prone to bloating**, repeat this remedy twice a day for five days, taking 1 drop of tarragon essential oil in 1 teaspoon of honey, between meals.

HEARTBURN

This is an unpleasant sensation of acidity in the digestive tract, which can sometimes feel like burning. It may be due to the reflux of stomach contents into the oesophagus (commonly known as acid reflux), but can also be caused by excess acidity or a particular sensitivity of the stomach wall. If you're prone to heartburn, start by improving your diet (an excess of sugar and fat encourages these symptoms) and making time to relax (stress is another aggravating factor). When heartburn is a particular problem, add these natural remedies.

BICARBONATE OF SODA (BAKING SODA)

It's simple, but very effective. Bicarbonate is a major antacid: you just need to swallow it to neutralize excess acidity.

TRY IT!
- **Pour ½ tablespoon** of bicarbonate of soda (baking soda) into a glass of water at room temperature.
- **Mix, and sip** as soon as you feel acidity or burning.
- **You can also** take bicarbonate of soda (baking soda) as a course of treatment: drink one glass a day for two weeks.

A LEMON INFUSION

The organic acids contained in lemon become alkalizing once in the stomach. They thus reduce the feeling of acidity and burning.

TRY IT!
- **Cut half an organic lemon** into thin slices. Put into a heat-proof container and add 200 ml (7 fl oz) of boiling water. Leave to cool to room temperature.
- **Filter, and drink** whenever you have heartburn.
- **You can also** take a lemon infusion cure by drinking a cup every morning, on an empty stomach before breakfast, for two weeks.

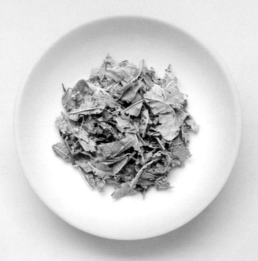

A LEMON VERBENA INFUSION

The lemon verbena plant, with its delicious citrus flavour, is antacid and carminative (it causes the expulsion of gas and relieves bloating), and aids digestion. It's also calming, which is helpful when heartburn is stress related.

TRY IT!
- **Add ½ tablespoon of the dried leaves** to a large cup of boiling water and leave to infuse for 5 minutes before filtering.
- **Drink a cup** after your two main meals, or whenever you're suffering from heartburn.

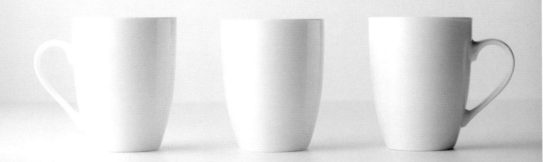

COLIC

The spasmodic intestinal pain associated with colic is often accompanied by diarrhoea. It's one of the manifestations of indigestion, but also of infectious gastroenteritis. These natural remedies can help to put an end to the stomach and intestine pain of colic.

BLACK TEA

You should avoid coffee when you have diarrhoea, but black tea is welcome because of its astringent properties. In addition, this drink helps to stop the spasms that make your belly painful.

TRY IT!

- **Prepare concentrated black tea** by pouring 1 tablespoon of tea leaves into a large cup of boiling water. Leave to steep for 10 minutes before filtering.
- **Drink three cups a day**, between meals, until the colic subsides.
- **Don't worry about the tea making you irritable or nervy:** the longer the infusion time, the more astringent tannins the leaves release, which neutralize the stimulant effect of the caffeine.

A DROP OF MARJORAM

This essential oil works wonders when the pain is a physiological reaction to a state of intense stress, or when fear (or another emotion) manifests itself as a pain in the stomach. As a bonus, marjoram is also a great digestion aid.

TRY IT!

- **Place only 1 drop** of marjoram essential oil on the tip of your tongue.
- **If the flavour is too strong for you**, you can dissolve it in ½ teaspoon of liquid honey. Keep it in your mouth for at least 10 seconds before swallowing.
- **Repeat** 4 hours later if symptoms persist.

A HAND MASSAGE

In the palm of the hand is an area corresponding to the intestine. Like the organ itself, this reflex zone is long. You'll therefore need to massage all along it to achieve a sufficient effect, but you can expect to see rapid results.

TRY IT!
- **Start by rubbing your hands together**, to warm them up.
- **Then, with the thumb of your right hand**, massage the palm of your left hand from the joint at the base of the thumb, towards the centre, then around the fleshy mound on the palm below the thumb, to return to the side of the wrist.
- **Massage for 2–3 minutes**, then do the same thing on the other hand.
- **Repeat** as often as necessary.

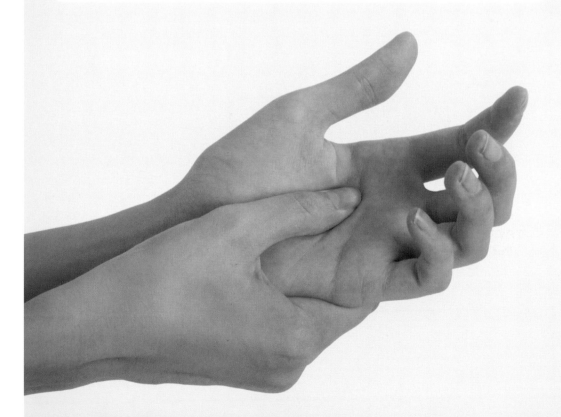

GASTRITIS

This is an inflammation of the stomach wall, which causes discomfort and can be very painful. To stop the pain, you'll need to calm the underlying inflammation. If the pain is incessant and becomes more intense, you should see a doctor. If it comes and goes, these few remedies can help to ease the problem.

A PLANT TO CHEW

Liquorice is anti-inflammatory, antispasmodic and antiulcerative – a winning combination for those who suffer from gastritis. In addition, it improves digestion. But be warned: avoid liquorice if you have high blood pressure, which it tends to raise.

TRY IT!
- **When you start to feel unwell**, chew a stick of liquorice root to extract the juice.
- **You can also** use liquorice powder (available in the baking section of some supermarkets), as long as it's not sweetened. Simply dissolve the powder in a glass of water.

A TURMERIC INFUSION

The anti-inflammatory properties of the turmeric spice make it ideal to consume as an infusion when you're suffering from gastritis – as well as using it in your cooking, of course!

TRY IT!
- **Put 1 level teaspoon of ground turmeric** in the bottom of a large cup and add a pinch of ground black pepper.
- **Add boiling water and leave to infuse for 10 minutes.** This is the time needed for the spice to diffuse its active components into the water and for the powder to settle at the bottom of the cup.
- **It's impossible to filter** this fine powder, so drink the infusion as it is, without stirring, so that you avoid swallowing the deposit that will have formed at the bottom of the cup.
- **Drink two cups a day**, after your main meals, for two weeks.

PAIN CHECKLIST: WHEN TO SEEK MEDICAL ADVICE

All these kinds of pain can be eased using the natural remedies covered in this book. There are times, though, when medical advice must be sought.

TYPE OF PAIN	POSSIBLE CAUSES	WHEN TO SEEK MEDICAL ADVICE
HEAD Throbbing pain, usually on one side of head	Migraine	Frequent and severe pain
MOUTH Pain in teeth	Toothache	Intense, throbbing pain that spreads to ear, jaw and neck; redness and swelling in face; shiny, red and swollen gums; sensitivity to hot or cold food and drink; fever; difficulty swallowing or breathing
Sores in mouth	Mouth ulcers	Ulcers that last for three weeks; frequently recurring ulcers; increased pain and redness
Red and swollen gums	Gingivitis	Bad breath; unpleasant taste in mouth; loose teeth; formation of abscesses
EAR, NOSE & THROAT Sharp, dull or burning ear pain	Earache	Fever; vomiting; severe sore throat; swelling around, or discharge from, ear
Pain when swallowing	Sore throat	No improvement after a week; difficulty breathing or swallowing; high-pitched sound when breathing
Pain, swelling and tenderness around cheeks, eyes or forehead	Sinusitis	No improvement after a week; frequently recurring symptoms
JOINT Pain in knee, shoulder or elbow	Tendinitis	No improvement within a few weeks; intense, sudden and severe pain
Throbbing and aching joint pain, swelling or stiffness – often worse in the morning	Rheumatoid arthritis Osteoarthritis	Always – to discover the underlying causes
Neck pain, which may travel down arm	Stiff neck	Numbness, pins and needles or weakness in one or both arms that gets worse; problems with balance or walking; blurred vision, ringing in ears or dizziness
Pain and discomfort between base of neck and top of hips	Back pain	Numbness or tingling around genitals or buttocks; difficulty passing water; loss of bladder or bowel control; chest pain; fever; unexplained weight loss; swelling in back

TYPE OF PAIN	POSSIBLE CAUSES	WHEN TO SEEK MEDICAL ADVICE
INJURY RELATED Pain following a bump	Haematoma (bruise) or contusion	No improvement within a couple of weeks; sudden onset of lots of bruises or bruising for no obvious reason
Soreness following exposure to sun	Sunburn	Blistering or swelling of skin; chills; fever; dizziness, headaches and feeling sick
Pain after exposing skin to strong heat source	Burns and scalds	All chemical and electrical burns; burns larger than a hand; white or charred skin; blisters on face, hands, arms, feet, legs or genitals
Pain around ankle, foot, wrist, thumb, knee, leg or back, with swelling and/or bruising	Sprain or strain	No improvement after self-treatment; worsening of pain or swelling; fever or feeling hot and shivery
CARDIOVASCULAR Pain in and around anus	Haemorrhoids (piles)	Persistent or severe pain; rectal bleeding
Aching, tender legs	Oedema (heavy legs)	Persistent pain; to check for potential underlying causes
FEMALE Pain in lower abdomen, possibly moving to lower back during a period	Painful menstruation	Severe period pains; changes in normal pattern of periods – for example, heavier than usual or more irregular
Dull, heavy or aching pain in breasts, sometimes spreading to armpits	Menstruation Sprains to neck, shoulder or back Pregnancy	No improvement after self-treatment; fever or feeling hot and shivery; red, hot or swollen breasts; family history of breast cancer; signs of pregnancy
DIGESTIVE Mild pain and sense of bloating in stomach area	Flatulence Bloating	Pain or bloating that won't go away or keeps coming back; repeated constipation or diarrhoea; unexpected weight loss; blood in stools; fever or feeling hot and shivery
Burning pain in middle of chest	Heartburn	Pain on most days for three weeks or more; food stuck in throat; frequent bouts of sickness; unexpected weight loss
Spasmodic intestinal pain, often with bloating and diarrhoea or constipation	Irritable bowel syndrome (IBS)	Unexpected weight loss; bleeding from bottom or bloody diarrhoea; hard lump or swelling in belly; shortness of breath, fast heart rate and pale skin
Gnawing or burning stomach pain	Gastritis	Symptoms that last a week or longer; severe pain; vomiting blood; blood in stools

QUICK-REFERENCE HERB & PLANT DIRECTORY

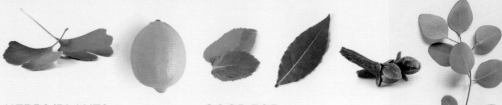

HERBS/PLANTS	GOOD FOR ...
Aloe vera	Burns and sunburn
Arnica	Bumps and bruises
Basil	Mouth ulcers
Bay leaf	Mouth ulcers
Blackcurrant	Stiff neck
Cabbage	Breast pains
Caraway	Flatulence
Chasteberry	Breast pains
Chilli	Small joints
Clove	Toothache
Cumin	Flatulence
Devil's claw	Rheumatic pain
Eucalyptus	Earache, sinus pain, large joints
Fennel	Flatulence
Feverfew	Headaches, period pains
Ginger	Flatulence
Gingko biloba	Haemorrhoids (piles)
Heather	Back pain
Helichrysum	Bumps and bruises, sprains
Horse chestnut bark	Heavy legs
Lavender	Stiff neck, burns and sunburn (lavender aspic essential oil)

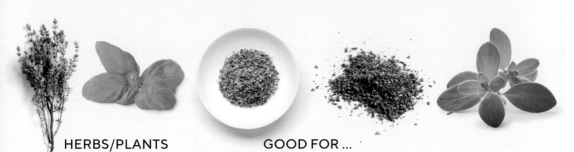

HERBS/PLANTS	GOOD FOR ...
Lemon	Mouth ulcers, large joints, bumps and bruises, heartburn
Lemon verbena	Heartburn
Liquorice	Gastritis
Marjoram	Colic
Mastic	Haemorrhoids (piles)
Meadowsweet	Headaches, rheumatic pain
Onion	Small joints
Peppermint	Headaches, gingivitis, rheumatic pain, sinus pain
Phytolacca (pokeweed)	Throat pain
Plum	Mouth ulcers
Rosemary	Muscle soreness and pain, stiff neck
St John's wort	Earache
Sweet clover	Heavy legs
Tarragon	Period pains, bloating
Tea	Colic
Thyme	Toothache, antiseptic mouthwash, sore throat
Turmeric	Gastritis
Willow bark	Tendinitis
Wintergreen	Tendinitis, rheumatic pain

NOTE: It's important to use a herb or plant in a form (such as oil, leaf or powder) that's safe and most effective for pain relief. Please see the specific herb and plant instructions given in the text for each treatment.

INDEX

PICTURE CREDITS

Front Cover
ShutterStockphoto.Inc (pill case) topseller; (pills top to bottom) matin, Kawongwarin, Fitria Ramli, JIANG HONGYAN, freya-photographer, Hans Christiansson, Alexander Ruiz Acevedo, Izf

Back Cover
ShutterStockphoto.Inc (pill case) topseller; (pills top to bottom) Africa Studio, Hong Vo, rodrigobark, Rtstudio, val lawless

ShutterStockphoto.Inc ShutterStockphoto.Inc 2 -3 Kerdkanno; 16-17 Dmitry Zimin; 21 Lisovskaya Natalia; 22 New Africa; 23 Jack Jelly; 24 StudioPhotoDFlorez; 25 sama_ja; 26, 27 StudioPhotoDFlorez; 28 Jack Jelly; 29 StudioPhotoDFlorez; 30 Charlotte Lake; 31 Michael Kraus; 32 artemisphoto; 33t StudioPhotoDFlorez; 33b Kiian Oksana; 34 StudioPhotoDFlorez; 35 margouillat photo; 36, 41 fizkes; 42 Image Point Fr; 44-5 fizkes; 48 mavo; 52 Elena Schweitzer; 53 Tatiana Kochkina; 54l matin; 54r drpnncpptak; 55, 56 Image Point Fr; 57 StudioPhotoDFlorez; 58 colorvsbw; 59t Nattika; 59b MaraZe; 60l EvilWata; 60r Viktor1; 61 VIRTEXIE; 62 Diana Taliun; 63 Madeleine Steinbach; 65 Upadhyay; 66 Dionisvera; 67 Image Point Fr; 69 Maren Winter; 70 Alexander Ruiz Acevedo; 72 file404; 73 Lukas Gojda; 74 Suto Norbert Zsolt; 75 RobsPhoto; 76 Image Point Fr; 77 Alim Yakubov; 79 TunedIn by Westend61; 80 Akvals; 81 Vladimir Gjorgiev; 82 MariaNikiforova; 83 PRO Stock Professional; 84 spline_x; 85 Comaniciu Dan; 86 Sakoodter Stocker; 87 LightField Studios; 88t BW Folsom; 88b hvoya; 89 Image Point Fr; 90 Elnur; 91 StudioPhotoDFlorez; 92 K.Decor; 94 PORNCHAI SODA; 95 Scisetti Alfio; 96 Carlo Zolesio; 97 Kotkoa; 98t ruangrit junkong; 98b Nenov Brothers Images; 100 Image Point Fr; 101 tulpahn; 103 nixki; 104 Peter Fuchs; 105 Masha_Semenova; 106t 12photography; 106b horiyan; 107 ShotPrime Studio; 108 ESB Professional; 109 Kaiskynet Studio; 110 ArtKio; 111l NAAN; 111r Ermak Oksana; 112l P-fotography; 112r COLOA Studio; 113 (left to right) Mny-Jhee, Viktor1, marilyn barbone; 114 StudioPhotoDFlorez; 115 Africa Studio; 116 OoddySmile Studio; 117 Slawomir Zelasko; 118t matin; 118b Shablon; 119 Hortimages; 120 Intarapong; 121 nito; 124 (left to right) nixki, StudioPhotoDFlorez, Africa Studio, MaraZe, Tim UR, K.Decor; 125 (left to right) StudioPhotoDFlorez, Volosina, matin, spline_x, Hortimages

ACKNOWLEDGEMENTS

Eddison Books Limited
Managing Director **Lisa Dyer**
Managing Editor **Tessa Monina**
Translation **Anne McDowall**
Designed and edited by **Fogdog Creative** (www.fogdog.co.uk)
Proofreader **Nikky Twyman**
Indexer **Marie Lorimer**
Production **Sarah Rooney & Cara Clapham**